ON A WING AND A PRAYER

Surviving a brain tumour

SARAH MY ANGEL, YOU WILL
ALWAYS HAVE MY LOVE

ON A WING AND A PRAYER
Surviving a brain tumour

Cameron Fulljames

JANUS PUBLISHING COMPANY
London, England

First published in Great Britain 2004
by Janus Publishing Company Ltd,
105-107 Gloucester Place,
London W1U 6BY

www.januspublishing.co.uk

British Library Cataloguing-in-Publication Data
A catalogue record for this book
is available from the British Library

ISBN 1 85756 578 9

Cover Design Simon Hughes

Printed and bound in Great Britain

For all my Heroes

Jamie (throat cancer), Cheryl and Pam (Hodgkin's lymphoma),
Paula and Graeme (brain tumours), Olivier (leukaemia),
Michael (prostate cancer) and in loving memory of my grandfather,
Raymond Fulljames (lung cancer), Peter Symes (bowel cancer) and
Andrew Schache (skin cancer).

Acknowledgements

I would like to thank my parents, Janet and Graham, and my partner, Sarah, for their unconditional love and support. Without their strength, I would have faced an impossible challenge. A special thanks to Eileen and Glenn, who helped make my book a reality. To Professor Ian Whittle, Professor Warnke, Dr Anna Gregor, Max, Shanne and the radiography team. There could never be words enough to express your gratitude to a group of people who have given you life. So let me just say – thank you.

Introduction

When I made the decision to record my thoughts in a diary, it was from a need to vent my frustration, anger, confusion and helplessness about what was happening to me. Reference material about brain tumour survivors was thin on the ground, with the result that I could never find answers that related to what I was experiencing.

Living with a brain tumour doesn't have to be about death, or slowly drifting into a void of dementia. It's about taking control and being positive. To me, there is nothing wrong with hope in the face of adversity and there is everything right with having a little optimism.

I hope this book goes some way to addressing these things. This is, simply, my story. In some small way it might help or comfort someone experiencing a similar illness – and the roller coaster ride that can go with it. At the very least, this is a story that was written in hope and which is about hope – as well as love, despair and, ultimately, survival.

From as far back as I can remember, I had wanted to fly aeroplanes. I was captivated by them and by those who flew them. Pilots were my heroes and mentors. From the Wright brothers to the Red Baron and from Douglas Bader to Chuck Yeager, I knew them all. They epitomised adventure, glamour and excitement – everything a young boy dreams of.

My father took me to every airshow around in my small home town of Tauranga, New Zealand. I can remember trembling with excitement as the A4 Skyhawks of the Royal New Zealand Air Force (RNZAF) did their flypast.

I was going to be a pilot; there was no question.

I built model aeroplanes and read every book I could find and even manipulated school project topics into aviation themes. "I wonder what your project will be about this time, Cameron," my teacher, Mrs Rewita, would say to me with a knowing smile.

My grandfather, who served in the RNZAF during World War II, and my parents, encouraged me. Dad took me for a trial flight at the local aero club when I was just eleven years old. Not young for a first flight, but young for flying lessons. I took these up immediately and paid for the lessons by doing odd jobs for neighbours. I would be airsick nearly every time, but I loved it. Flying was the ultimate freedom. It was a sense of space and exhilaration. Nothing compared.

5 July, 2000

The 5th of July, 2000, was a day that was to change my life forever, in ways I could never have imagined. Everything would undergo a major shift, from the security of my career to the good health that I, like so many, took for granted.

I awoke to be confronted by two paramedics. They were asking me questions, and I felt dazed. Something had happened but I didn't know what. I was confused yet coherent and could see Sarah in the background. She looked worried, a little frantic. The paramedics moved me to a stretcher and took me to an ambulance waiting outside.

When I had first met Sarah three months previously she was walking down the steps of a nightclub towards me. I watched transfixed: I'd never seen a woman so beautiful. Everything about her seemed so perfect and wonderful. I fell in love immediately. I hadn't been looking for a relationship, let alone love, but in that moment she stole my heart forever. I knew I never wanted to be without this person.

As she walked past I grabbed her. I couldn't speak, but... She looked at me, not attempting to break free

"Would you like a drink?" I stammered. It was neither original nor romantic, but it was the best I could do under the circumstances.

"Yes," she replied.

In the following months, we had a whirlwind romance, including a ten-day holiday in Greece. On the morning after our flight back to the United Kingdom, I drove from Newcastle to Edinburgh, collected my belongings, cleaned the flat and then drove to Sarah's family home in Forfar. I was being re-based to Aberdeen, one of three Scottish bases my airline operated out of. Base changes for aircrew were rare but necessary so to ensure there were enough crew could cover the flight schedule, and had left everything to the last minute. It had been a long day and that evening, I was feeling a little nauseous. I put it down to tiredness and decided to have an early night.

12 July, 2000

My appointment with Dr Rutherford seemed routine enough. In fact,

I was keen to get some answers as to why I'd had this seizure. My opinion was that it had been caused by stress and fatigue after my holiday and base change. I was looking for support and some confirmation of that.

I'd not had an EEG (electroencephalogram) before, but knew it was something I had to pass. It was a Civil Aviation Authority test that my flying career depended upon.

The EEG was conducted by a nurse. A number of receptors were stuck to my skull, followed by a series of tests involving flickering lights. A junior doctor then gave me a neurological examination. I wondered at this – my career was at stake, and I wanted an expert to examine me and give the verdict.

But all seemed well, and a short time later I was called in for a consultation with Dr. Rutherford.

"You have epilepsy," he said simply. "You experienced a classic tonic-clonic seizure."

This threw me into a state of shock. I knew only too well what impact this would have on my flying career. So did Sarah, who held tightly onto my hand.

As Dr Rutherford continued to talk, all I could think about was how he had not interviewed me on the events leading up to the seizure. He didn't even examine me. Who did he think he was, basing his opinion simply on the seizure type?

"You are obligated to inform the DVLA [Driver & Vehicle Licensing Agency]," Dr Rutherford continued, "who will suspend your licence. You cannot drive and it is up to you to inform whomever the controlling authority is about your flying licence. This is your responsibility, but can I just say that if it were you who were piloting the aircraft I was getting on, I wouldn't fly with you."

I couldn't believe what was being said to me. How could he challenge my integrity? Sarah and I looked at each other in dismay. She gripped my arm.

"You will need to have an MRI scan," concluded Dr Rutherford. "One has been booked for you in three months' time – it's quite routine."

An MRI scan in three months? I didn't have time for that! I needed to get this matter behind me and get back into the air. I was thirty years old and being told I had epilepsy. I'd never heard anything more ridiculous. I needed a second opinion, someone who could talk some sense to me... Dr Brooker? I knew and trusted him. Yes, he would help.

Extract taken from: *Epilepsy Ontario.*
In a generalized tonic-clonic (grand mal) seizure, the person will usually emit a short cry and fall to the floor. Their muscles will stiffen (tonic phase) and then their extremities will jerk and twitch (clonic phase). Bladder control may be lost. Teeth may be clenched and frothing at the mouth may occur. Consciousness is regained slowly.

After a seizure, the person may feel fatigue, confusion and disorientation. This may last from 5 minutes to several hours or even days. Rarely, this disorientation may last up to 2 weeks. The person may fall asleep, or gradually become less confused until full consciousness is regained.

Dr Brooker had always put me at ease. An elderly, distinguished gentleman, he'd done two of my previous CAA medicals and had been around aviation a long time.

"So Cameron, what are you calling this episode?" he asked. "A faint, fit, turn or seizure?"

"Seizure," I replied. "Fit" sounded too much like epilepsy and "a turn" was something old people had.

Dr Brooker knew how damning Sarah's recollection of the seizure was, and he began questioning her. He's on my side, I thought.

I gave my medical history and some background to the seizure, then Dr Brooker concluded with, "Alcohol withdrawal." Sounded plausible to me.

***

I continued to live with Sarah's family in Scotland. Her parents, David and Lynda, were in their early fifties and her younger brother and sister, Michael and Rachael, still lived at home. I loved being there, immersed in a family environment. It was something I hadn't experienced in a long time.

13 July, 2000

I went to the library to get some books on epilepsy. As I read, something alarmed me, sending a shiver through my body. The most likely cause of epilepsy in patients with a first-time seizure after the age of thirty is a brain tumour. This frightened me. Not only had I just had a first-time seizure, but I was also thirty. God! Do I have a brain tumour?

With my career in jeopardy due to the epilepsy diagnosis, I needed the help of a specialist. I approached my employer for the assistance of the company's medical insurance and was able to book a consultant immediately.

14 July, 2000

I received a letter from the CAA advising me that I had been assessed as temporarily unfit to hold a pilot's licence of any kind.

27 July, 2000

The appointment with a new consultant was booked: I was excited that today I'd get some serious answers about the future of my career! But I was also nervous. What if the neurologist didn't concur with the over-tired, alcohol withdrawal theory? I'll just get another opinion, I thought defiantly.

I arrived in Edinburgh and entered a very plush reception room, thinking I was glad I wasn't paying for the consultation.

Dr Colin Mumford strolled out to greet me and I shook his hand. He looked young, about my age, and that immediately put me at ease. I could relate to him and, as he began the examination, he seemed to be on my side.

Colin told me that he was attached to the CAA and knew the chap who'd be examining me at Gatwick. The neurology exam was as I'd already experienced, and in the following interview he seemed to agree with Dr Brooker's reason for my seizure.

At last someone was making sense, and taking an interest in me and my career. Colin said that I should get my medical back, and that he would personally recommend it – pending an MRI scan, of course.

"When can I get an MRI done?" I asked. "Ninewells Hospital have booked one for me but not until October."

Colin made a call to the Western General Hospital and got me in – for that afternoon! The excitement rushed through me. It was all happening. I was going to get my medical back – and with it, the life that I adored.

I had some time to kill so I e-mailed Mum and Dad from a nearby Internet café.

The e-mail:
A wee poem about being a 'kiwi'.
"Call me an epileptic, clip my wings, and cause me dismay.
But I'm a 'kiwi', born to fly; you're not taking my medical away!"

So much has happened this week, I don't know where to start. Yes, I do. How are you all, good?

Monday I posted a message on the Internet with an airline pilots' site asking if anyone else in the UK had suffered a similar problem to myself. A chap e-mailed me that he had had a seizure and got his medical back.

The CAA medical advisor phoned me and gave me a run through on the process of dealing with my medical. Great – at least someone down there cares.

Binned the idiot who initially called me an epileptic and went private, finding a consultant who by chance happens to be with the CAA.

Today (Fri) had the consultation with this doctor, who was superb, was very sympathetic and said I am not an epileptic, but had a "one-off" seizure brought on by sleep deprivation. Bloody fantastic; at last someone is talking some sense!!!!!!!!!!!! Quick as a flash he organised an MRI scan this afternoon. I am in Edinburgh, by the way. Appointment is booked with CAA med advisor on 8 Sept 00. This guy has the ultimate decision. But my guy knows him and he will be making a recommendation to him. Hope that all makes sense. RING ME!!!!!!!!

I miss Sarah desperately, have bonded with Michael and have a little brother to look after. Sarah's parents have been amazing.

A command is awaiting me when I return to flying. Yeeha!!!!

Must go (I'm in an Internet café)

Take care,

Love, Cam

I arrived at the Department of Clinical Neurosciences that afternoon and took a seat in the waiting room. There were a lot of people already waiting and, as I looked around, the scars and the signs of brain surgery soon became evident. I felt uncomfortable.

I sat opposite a young couple who both looked vacant and radiated a type of sadness which said, "There is nothing left to do but die, the fight has left us." I watched her clutch his arm.

My name was called and I was shown into the MRI waiting room. I'd seen MRI scans before in magazines, and this didn't look as threatening as I had thought. Colin had arrived and he gave me a wave.

I was instructed to remove any metallic objects, and as I was doing so was given a choice of music – Barry Manilow or Queen. I laughed, and answered, "Queen, please." I was given the dos and don'ts and the nurse finished by saying, "It'll be all over in about fifteen minutes."

I felt claustrophobic as my upper body entered the tubular structure. I was kept informed of the scan's progress through my headphones, which had the annoying result of periodically cutting out the song I was listening to. I started to feel a little strange, so focused on a point above me, and I sang to the beat of *Bohemian Rhapsody*.

I was pulled out and greeted by a surgeon. Complete with green pyjamas and hat, he was holding a very large needle that looked like it was intended for me. "I'm just going to give you a small injection," he said. "This material makes the scan a little clearer."

The sequence of scans was repeated. Something was wrong, I knew it. What was supposed to take fifteen minutes had now taken half an hour. I listened to the music and tried to relax.

When it was over I returned to the waiting room and dressed myself. As I sat there, Colin entered the room.

"Well, fuck me!" he exclaimed. "I'm gobsmacked. You've got a brain tumour!"

Before I had a chance to contemplate what he'd said, Colin sat down and explained what the MRI had found. As he showed me the tumour on the X-ray, I felt a strange sense of relief. Relief because I could now physically see what had caused the seizure, I wasn't going mad, nor did I have epilepsy. In an odd sort of way, I felt smug.

But the tumour was huge. It occupied what appeared to me to be a quarter of my brain. Colin said that he would ask a surgeon to come and talk to me, and I was asked to take a seat in the main waiting room. "They'll only be five minutes," he said, "and she's one of the best. I'll see you soon."

When I returned to the waiting room, it was empty apart from the couple I'd seen earlier. She gave me the same vacant look, sensing my result but sharing no emotion.

As I sat waiting, I recalled the only person I'd ever known to have a brain tumour. It was a woman I met in a naval hospital in New Zealand. She had lived out her last years in a gradual, downward spiral of dementia and loneliness.

I stood up and moved towards the main doors, fumbling a cigarette to my lips. I felt so alone. I needed to talk to someone. A friend, any friend.

JD came first to mind, but there was no answer. Francis – no answer. Hamish – no answer. Please, somebody!

Hilton answered, thank God. (Hilton was an old friend from my years at boarding school.) I dribbled information to him, probably making no sense. All I could hear was his calm, controlled voice: "I'm coming up to see you. It's okay mate, I'm coming up."

I went back inside to find the waiting room empty and sat down. A nurse walked past me. "Can I get you a coffee or tea?" The way she said it sounded as if she were saying, "I'm sorry."

"Coffee, please," I replied.

After what seemed like an eternity, Dr Lynn Moore entered with five or six junior doctors in tow. They sat in a semicircle in front of me, all in white coats. This scared me – I felt like I was at a job interview, or worse, in a mental hospital!

Dr Moore was certain of the tumour I had and how advanced it was. I was bombarded with medical jargon I didn't understand, and then she spoke of how I only had five years to live, but that they were going to prolong my life.

As she spoke, I seemed to drift away. I couldn't take it all in. I had never felt more alone in all my life. I sat like a frightened child, and when she left, Colin's comforting smile greeted me. Just for a moment, I felt everything was going to be okay. But it wasn't.

I needed to go. I got into my car and headed home. I needed to be surrounded by people I knew and who knew me. As I drove, I mulled over what Dr Moore had said. Five years is all I have to live, I thought. Just five years. And then I remembered Sarah. How would I tell my Sarah?

When I arrived home, I walked into the kitchen and stared at David and Lynda, motioning for David to join me outside. I sat on the deckchair and David sat opposite. "I have a brain tumour." I paused, then said, "I'm scared, really scared." I felt Lynda's arms encircle me from behind. I could hear her crying. David moved closer, and rubbed my shoulder.

The MRI had shown a large infiltrative tumour in the temporal lobe. It was turning malignant and would need immediate treatment.

28 July, 2000

I broke down and wept as I have never wept before. In my adult life I had only ever cried twice. The first was when my first love, Kate Jackson, broke up with me. The second was when my great uncle died.

I was only thirty years old and I was going to die. I was scared and confused. Why had God forsaken me? I thought about my life. I'd had two careers, and achieved my goals in both. I had been married and separated. What was left to do? Was this my whack? Was this it?

***

As soon as I was old enough I'd applied to be a fighter pilot in the Royal New Zealand Air Force. Failing the selection process, I was devastated. But at seventeen years old, I was really too young and lacked the maturity required for the armed services. So I left high school and took a year out, travelling around New Zealand and working in various labouring jobs in the building industry. Returning to Auckland, I joined the Royal New Zealand Navy as a seaman officer. But after four years' service, the call to flying became too strong and I resigned to pursue my flying career.

Looking back, at this time in my life I had spent eleven years in institutions, starting with boarding school at thirteen until I left the Navy in 1995. As a consequence, I'd become very independent from a young age and my relationship with my family had suffered. Unknowingly, I had continued to distance myself from them right up until I flew out to the United Kingdom.

My decision to move to the United Kingdom was directly related to the poor job prospects for commercial pilots in New Zealand at the time. I had been working as a flight instructor at a local flying school and also as a commercial pilot for an aerial surveying company. But there was just no money in it. The flying I had done in N.Z. had been fabulous, but after five years it was time to move on to the big jets

29 July, 2000
Sarah arrived home after flying back early from a pilgrimage to Lourdes. I met her at the airport and we hugged. I was going to need her like I had never needed anyone before. I wondered if this tumour were fate. I knew that I was strong enough to cope. I found solace by concluding that if tumours really do occur randomly, then it was better that I dealt with it rather than a small child or someone less able to cope.

I was going to have to heal my brain through natural healing. The human body has an amazing ability to heal itself, and the power of the mind is the catalyst. It was all up to me. I knew it!

1 August, 2000
My sister, Anna, rang. "Is it a glioblastoma?" she asked.

"Yes," I lied, having no idea what a glioblastoma was. I didn't even know if my tumour as, malignant or benign.

Shortly after my conversation with Anna, Mum and Dad phoned to say they were coming over. I was angry with Anna as she'd obviously put the fear of God into our parents. I needed to be in control. I could look after myself! What I wanted was my life back, to feel normal. I worried that, with my parents here, I'd be constantly reminded that things weren't right. I needed my independence, yet it was about to be taken away.

Dr. Moore had asked me to come back on the 4th of August for a biopsy and to talk with her further about the tumour. I rang Hilton and, before I could finish telling him about the biopsy, he said he was coming with me and would be on the next flight to Edinburgh. This time I was relieved. I had no choice in the matter, and the fact was I was going to need him.

I'd begun to shut down and close off to people near to me, something that had always been my natural defence mechanism. I didn't want sympathy, or people to treat me differently. So, as work colleagues and friends found out about my condition, I unknowingly distanced myself by making it known that I didn't want their sympathy. This was hard for them; they had difficulty knowing just how to approach me. The result was that many never contacted me at all. It was one of the many lessons about myself I was to learn in the coming months.

3 August, 2000

I felt that I needed to go to church. I asked Sarah if she would come with me. David drove us to an Anglican church that was opened especially for us. Whether it was a need for some divine inspiration or just to be somewhere that was peaceful and reassuring to contemplate things, I don't know. But I prayed like I had never prayed before.

4 August, 2000

Lynda, Sarah and I went to pick up Hilton from the airport.

As we walked through one of the neurosurgery wards looking for Dr Moore, we could see some of the patients. The scars, the vacant looks, the signs of dementia... It was horrible.

Dr Moore led us into a store cupboard, of all places, to talk. There were no chairs, so we all stood. "The professor's away at the moment," she said, "but I can do your biopsy this afternoon if you like."

I was confused. Here I was being given a decision to make with absolutely no idea of what a biopsy was. I didn't know anything about its importance, the risks or even the options.

"No," Hilton replied emphatically. "We'll wait for Professor Whittle."

I sighed with relief, relief that I didn't have to make the decision.

Hilton had asked all the questions and had made a judgement call that later proved to have been the right one.

7 August, 2000

I moved back to Edinburgh with Mum and Dad and we rented a flat. I wrote in my diary, "How did my life come to this? In Edinburgh with my parents, living with people I don't know, driving me mad. I don't need this constant reminder of my illness. I need to get out; where's [my friend] JD?"

10 August, 2000

I had my second seizure. As I lay in bed asleep, somewhere between consciousness and unconsciousness, I could hear myself snoring. When I came to, Mum and Dad were lying beside me, comforting me. I sat up to find my shoulders and joints aching. I felt drowsy and a little nauseous – these were to become the calling cards of my seizures.

Unknown to me at the time, Mum and Dad had sought help from the Cancer Support Group. This is their story.

Brain tumour. The very words conjure up nightmares of seizures, paralysis, loss of sight, memory, intellect, and finally death. Our beautiful son, an airline pilot. This news was surely more than my husband and I could bear. It's not happening; don't tell anyone; perhaps the diagnosis is wrong. Try not to show any emotion on the phone. Don't convey anxiety; leap on the first plane to Edinburgh. We were there in three days.

The biggest problem was that Cameron's specialist had left for a conference in the United States and we had to wait six weeks for an appointment. So there was no one of whom we could ask questions, and we were faced with a son who was very much in denial.

Remain calm! Go through the motions of eating, sleeping and trying to find accommodation during the Edinburgh Festival. Our New Zealand dollar was three point three to one against us and we were in the United Kingdom for the long haul. But much worse than that was a grieving son with his career in tatters.

Soon after we arrived, Cameron had his second seizure at 6.00am one morning. Suddenly he was just three years old again and needing help. Graham and I lay with him, protecting him until the seizure passed and he gained consciousness. What was happening to him? No one to ask! Finally, after the third seizure, we tried to seek help. We phoned someone whose name and number we found in a brochure on brain tumours. We hid this from Cameron, as he emphatically did not want to talk to other brain tumour victims at this stage. (Keeping in mind that we did not know precisely what tumour he had.)

Yes! A very nice woman took our call and we arranged to meet in the foyer of the Caledonian Hotel, a landmark in Edinburgh, but a very austere atmosphere for the warm, positive chat we were expecting. We needed practical help, reassurance, warmth, a shoulder to cry on – and most of all, hope.

Instead, what we met was austerity, formality and a formidable person. She had survived her brain tumour, certainly, but in her words, "feared waking up every morning in case her tumour had returned." After seven years in full recovery, she had become a control freak and her first words to us were, "Welcome to the nightmare of the brain tumour. I know a thirty year-old who lived for three years after his diagnosis."

She might as well have said, "It's your turn to walk the plank!" I gripped Graham's hand, with tears flowing uncontrollably. "It's okay, you're in shock," she said kindly. "And perhaps find a B&B for your accommodation – it'll be cheaper."

A B&B with our son having seizures every week? We left hurriedly with a pile of pamphlets and a quick "don't call us; we'll call you!" We both looked at one another outside the hotel. That had been a big mistake.

To be fair, there was one piece of advice we were given that day that will forever stick in our minds. "He's a pilot so the best thing for him to do is stay in the industry. If he focuses on getting back in the air, it is his best chance for recovery."

14 August, 2000
I had been giving my future a great deal of thought. It was part of my plan to get better. There were three things I needed to do to take control:

- One, to be in Edinburgh, a city that I adored and where I'd be close to Sarah.
- Two, to be surrounded by positive people.
- Three, I had to find a career that was as stimulating to me as my flying.

The last one was going to be the hardest. My only two interests outside aviation that were potential careers were photography and archaeology. I began to make enquires about archaeology at Edinburgh University but had to abandon the idea as I'd not undertaken any previous university study in the United Kingdom.

My application was rejected and I wrote in my diary, "Archaeology, no places this year. God, will I ever start getting a change of fortune? I need to start taking charge of my own career moves and destiny. I must take responsibility for myself. I feel terrible for the way I have treated Mum and Dad; I miss them."

15 August, 2000

Francis (a colleague from British Midland) sent me a text message, So what's the long-term prognosis?" I texted back, "The day I live my life to a time frame will be the day I die." He didn't answer.

17 August, 2000

I wrote two words in my diary: "Courageous" and "Passionate." These were what I believed I was going to need to be.

Skim-reading through a book on brain tumours from the medical library, I found most of the statistics and words confusing. However, one passage jumped out at me: 20,000 people are diagnosed with gliomas in the U.S.A. each year; half die within eighteen months.

I stared blankly at this statement, and then in a tidal wave of want, aggression and desire for life, I hatched my plan: a plan to fight this disease, the intruder into my life.

My eight-stage plan:
- I would live in Edinburgh, the city I adored.
- I would buy a house to maintain my independence.
- I would pursue a new career and continue to work my brain mentally by doing crosswords, puzzles and the like.
- Remove all stresses in my life and ensure I got quality sleep.
- I would get advice on nutrition and eat healthily.
- I would remain fit but avoid any exercise that might increase cranial pressure.
- I would empower myself through knowledge and read everything I could about my tumour and the treatments available.
- I would remain in control; the tumour would not control me.

23 August, 2000

This was the day I signed up for photography at the college. I had been running around in circles about the future. Photography was my second love, but would it give me the satisfaction flying did? I knew that it was unlikely, but I had to do something.

Photography was to fill a void over the coming months. Through it I was able to be creative and express myself in ways I'd never done before. Time in the darkroom was a period of calm for me. I was doing some good work and, for a while, I was proud of myself and excited.

30 August, 2000

My consultation with Professor Whittle was at 3.00pm. What he was going to say would have a huge bearing on my future. He had the experience and the answers.

Mum, Dad and Sarah were with me. As we walked into the room, we saw a young guy, not the grey-haired gentleman you might associate with the title "professor." His head was evenly shaved and I admired his attempt to empathise with his patients. Whittle had a deep Australian accent, and it gave me comfort to know that a fellow Antipodean was helping me (even if he was an Australian!).

My parents were desperate to hear something positive and they weren't disappointed. The first thing Professor Whittle talked about was an operation. He said there was a surgeon in America who had perfected a technique of resecting infiltrative brain tumours, which were normally inoperable. This surgeon had performed the operation over a hundred times, with a 95% success rate.

We learnt that being able to operate and resect all, or most, of the tumour plays a pivotal role in the life span and health of a patient. The difficulty with a temporal lobe tumour is that it encompasses the cerebral artery, making total resection dangerous and almost impossible.

It was reassuring to know that they could operate. He went on to say that radiotherapy would be the first treatment because it was safe and they knew it worked.

I wanted a prognosis and asked the question, How long did I have to live? The professor shrugged it off quickly and replied, "Ask me again when you're seventy, Cameron."

"You mean he will live to an old age?" my mother asked excitedly.

"Of course, madam. There is not a disease, illness or cancer on this planet that somebody hasn't made a full recovery from, and that includes full-blown AIDS."

The mood in the room had changed completely. The positivity was electric. My mother needed to hear these words. When we left the room Sarah's arms engulfed me from behind. I was grateful to Professor Whittle; he had given my family hope. He did more for me with the words he spoke that day than he could have ever done with his hands and a scalpel.

I would often sit in the garden with a lit cigarette and gaze at the night sky, waiting for the Aberdeen-to-Edinburgh night mail run to pass overhead. Clear, still, cold nights always reminded me of night mails. I loved to fly at night when you could look at the maze of city lights emerging from the horizon and see the stars above you. So peaceful. Just me, the aeroplane and two tonnes of mail. I missed flying.

4 September, 2000

Mum gave me a book that was to become my bible. It was called *Love, Medicine and Miracles*, by Bernie Seigel. As I read, I noted the following passage, "Demand dignity, personhood and control no matter what the course of the disease. It takes courage to be exceptional."

These words rang in my brain. "It takes courage to be exceptional" became the code I lived by throughout the coming months. I wanted to be exceptional!

The next day, JMC airlines called me for interview. It was my dream job. A medium haul out of Glasgow – a base I wanted because it meant being close to Sarah. Flying a Boeing 757, I could fulfil a dream of flying a wide-body jet, and earning great money. I explained my situation to the recruiting representative and reluctantly declined the interview. I was disappointed. That afternoon I noted from my "bible", "In the face of uncertainty, there is nothing wrong with hope."

6 September, 2000

The JMC interview played on my mind, and affected me more than I thought. I was deeply disappointed.

12 September, 2000
Our offer on the flat in Edinburgh was accepted. Yeeha! Phases one and two of my plan were in place.

13 September, 2000
My close friend JD called me. JD was like the older brother I'd never had, and he said, "Cam, you're a pilot, and you'll always be a pilot." His words made me feel better and I wrote them in my diary, in bold.

22 September, 2000
I was on the way to do some shopping with Mum and Dad when Declan Dooney rang. Declan was the recruiting officer for Ryanair, an airline I'd been trying to get into for at least two years. No first officers had been taken in that time, yet here he was, ringing to invite me to an interview. This was my lowest point. I felt as if somebody was deliberately trying to kick me in the teeth. *Why Does it Always Rain on me?* by Travis played on the radio. I needed Sarah.

The renovations on my flat had drained me financially and Dad was also feeling the pinch, so I took a job as a barman at a pub in town. £4.00 an hour plus tips wasn't bad, and Dad welcomed the money.

6 October, 2000
My chief pilot, Captain Paul Yarnold, rang. He asked me how I was and we talked about my treatment. He finished the conversation by saying, "Cameron, Midland sell jumpseat rides to raise money for charity. Hell, if we do it for others we can do it for you!"

I was humbled: it was one of the kindest gestures anyone had ever offered me. Paul rang many times, along with another senior captain, Frank Brown. Frank had returned to flying after losing a leg in an air accident. Typically Irish, with the fiery temper of a Celt and a razor-sharp wit, he was my mentor and gave me much of my inspiration to get well.

23 October, 2000

I received notification of my biopsy. It was scheduled for the 3rd of November.

I couldn't help but feel sad. I'd just started to forget about the tumour and had been getting on with my life. Photography was proving to be something I was good at and enjoyed, and the building work on the house was going well and nearing completion.

I sat down at the kitchen table to write my will. I really had no rationale for this, except that the professor's admission that there was a 5% chance that the biopsy could go wrong had really got to me.

As I wrote, leaving possessions to friends and relatives, I started to feel sad. The more I wrote, the sadder I got. Feeling engulfed by my grief I stood up and walked off. I couldn't take it any more.

"Where are you going, mate?" Dad asked.

"Going for a run."

I needed to blow off some steam. It had started to rain outside, but I needed to go. I needed to see Sarah; a moment with her always made my troubles fade away. She was my link to my former life. When I was with her I felt wonderful. I adored her.

It was raining heavily when I kissed Sarah goodbye and began my run home. I was exhausted by the time I finally drifted off to sleep.

In the early hours of the following morning, I had another seizure, but this time I had convulsed out of bed. Mum and Dad found me on the floor. I came to as Mum rubbed my back. I had a carpet burn down one side of my face and a bump on my forehead where I had hit the side-table. Looking in the mirror, I wondered how I was going to explain my injuries to the bar staff, my photography course mates, and especially to Sarah.

30 October, 2000 (Monday)

The charge nurse showed me to my room. She was a well-built woman in her sixties and what she said was gospel. God help anyone who dared question her, but she had a heart of gold. I had a long wait to see the professor who would be doing my surgery, and a string of doctors visited me over the next two hours.

The first specialist I met was an Australian pharmacist. Another Antipodan involved in my treatment! Was this being done on purpose to ease my concerns?

In addition to prescribing the medication I was going to need, he gave me a thorough run-down on my operation. He mentioned I'd be on a course of steroids, to reduce the brain swelling. My eyes lit up. Anabolic steroids? I wondered. Maybe the effects of the steroids could be put to good use in the gym before they wore off... He noticed my interest and said with a smile, "No, not anabolic steroids!"

The professor entered. A capable, intelligent-looking gentleman, he spoke with a staunch German accent. His time was precious and he was only with me briefly. He outlined the day of surgery and explained that the irregularity in my brain was either 98% tumour or 2% inflammation. "Give me the 2%," I said. I was in good hands; I liked him.

After eating my corned beef hash, I tracked down the smokers' room. Inside the room, amongst a cloud of smoke and the stale smell of tobacco, were Sharon, Mary and Tony. Tony was in his early sixties but looked twenty years younger. He wore shorts and a T-shirt and gave the impression he'd just been out for a run. As I entered the room, they were in full discussion. It appeared Sharon had constipation. "The steroids will cause this," said Mary. Tony retorted, "All you need is a spoon that'll get the hard bit out." I raised my eyebrows and smiled at Tony. He obviously enjoyed his conversations with the girls. Sharon continued, "It's my period at the moment. I'm bunged up in the rear and I'm bunged up in the front."

On that note I made a hasty exit. I'd heard enough!

31 October, 2000 (Tuesday)

I spoke to Mary that afternoon while having a smoke. Mary was in her late sixties and looked it, probably due to years of smoking and gin drinking. Her tumour had spread to her brain from another cancer in her body. She took pride in telling me that the tumour had a tail on it. The mental picture of a tumour with a tail gave it an evil identity, so I just nodded and changed the subject. She was a strong person and I admired her fight. I got up to leave, picking up a newspaper as I walked out. "Good luck, love!" she bellowed.

1 November, 2000 (Wednesday)
The pre-op team came earlier than expected. I wasn't prepared. During the morning, I'd become increasingly relaxed about it all. I was looking forward to the first stage of treatment and recovery. As I removed my bracelet, I could feel Sarah behind me and heard her crying.

"Find an eyelash so I can make a wish," I said. She smiled. I could see Mum crying. I choked a little. The staff nurse noticed the tears and commanded, "That will be enough of that!"

We approached the surgery doors and stopped. I pulled Sarah towards me and had just enough time to whisper, "I love you."

In the anaesthetic room, the nurses joked. They were a lovely group of women, who immediately put me at ease, and I laughed with them. The local anaesthetic injections in my forehead were painful. A nurse held my hand, making me feel more relaxed.

I'd been asked whether I'd like to be sedated or have local anaesthetic followed by sedation, or just receive local anaesthetic only. I replied, "What's more painful, childbirth or a biopsy?"

"Childbirth," replied the professor.

"Just a local then," I said. I was determined to stay awake throughout the operation; it was about being in control of what was happening to me. I was petrified of waking up with brain damage.

The halo was fitted. The screws into my forehead were excruciating. I could feel my skin squish and twist as the screw was turned. Then came the pressure on my skull – it was almost unbearable. As I relaxed my head back on the pillow the rear screws dug in and I cringed. Then the local finally kicked in, and I relaxed. I was then whisked off to the MRI scanner, although this time I knew what to expect. It only took four minutes – no problem!

As my eyes went in and out of focus, I wiggled my feet and sang, *You've Lost that Loving Feeling* to stay alert. It was the only song that I knew in its entirety, thanks to my Navy days.

Once in the theatre, my anxiety came back. The prof. marked out the area of entry and a nurse started to shave. I couldn't believe it: she was dry-shaving my head! I told her that it was the most painful part of the operation so far, which was the first time I'd mentioned any discomfort. A little anaesthetic was used as a lubricant, and thankfully offered some relief.

I heard a nurse say, "Doesn't he look like Liam Neeson," and thought how appalled Mr. Neeson would be to hear that compliment, given the state I was in!

An incision was made and my skin was clamped back. A painful, stinging sensation began, which lasted for the entire operation. I felt nothing as the professor commenced drilling a hole into my skull, about the size of a tenpence. There was no activity, just the sound, which differed from the high-pitched whirring of a dentist's drill that I'd imagined. Suddenly the drill bit grabbed and jerked my head around violently. I squeezed the nurse's hand. "Shit!" I gasped.

The professor apologised and switched to a hand drill. This seemed to take an eternity. "You should stop using the drill bits for your own DIY," I said. He laughed.

I felt an increased weight pushing down on the drill. All I could think of was the drill suddenly bursting through my skull and lodging itself into my brain... I continued to breathe deeply and wiggle my feet. When the hole was finally opened, I can't think of a moment when I've been more relieved.

Several samples were to be taken and, as I lay there, I began to think how amazing the situation was. "This is outrageous!" I exclaimed as the prof. moved the probe in and out of my brain. Here I was, fully conscious with a hole in my skull, while a probe was being inserted in my brain. It was almost crude, like an operation with saws and large blunt instruments from hundreds of years ago. But it was also fantastic!

I couldn't resist asking, "What colour is it?"

"What?" the nurse replied.

"My brain," I said

"What colour is it?"

"A grey, greeny colour," she replied in a bemused voice.

As the last sample was taken, relief washed over me and I longed for them to remove that horrible head brace.

Recovery took an hour and by then I was desperate for a cigarette. Kath, the ward sister, came and spoke to me. She had a wonderful warm manner about her and we spoke for the whole hour, mainly about her fear of flying. It was some much-needed company.

I longed for Sarah; I longed to show her how well I was. I was proud of myself. I hadn't used a sedative and had endured the pain. The hour quickly passed and I was soon heading back to the ward, this time to a room with guys my own age.

I sat up in bed, needing that cigarette. I felt okay so I swung my legs off the end of the bed. But I was entangled in the line of the saline drip. I'll take that with me, I thought, although getting dressed was no easy task.

I made my way out of the ward into the corridor, only to be confronted by the staff nurse. "And where do you think you're going?" she glared.

I didn't reply, instead turning and making my way back to the ward, drip in hand. Damn! I wanted a good reason why I was bed-ridden, deprived of cigarettes, food and drink. When the ward was quiet again, I got up and had a cigarette in the adjacent ward toilet. I was a terrible patient in recovery, stubborn to the end.

The professor saw me during his evening rounds and commented, "He looks healthy apart from his nicotine and caffeine addictions." I noticed his blue tie dotted with little yellow teddy bears and retorted, "Nice tie!"

I detected relief in his eyes and body language. It occurred to me how much pressure he must be under during surgery – especially surgery involving the brain, where a small mistake could mean a huge price to pay. The professor explained that they had gone deep into my brain, hence I needed to stay in bed for a period because there was fear of collapse if I were to stand up. It was a good enough reason for me and I finally behaved. I negotiated a cappuccino with the professor. Mum brought me two!

Later that evening, an understanding sister freed me of the drip and

I fled to the smokers' room. I found Sharon alone in the room, her forehead resting on the palm of her hand. I sat down beside her.

Sharon was a few years older than I and slightly overweight. She was awaiting the results of her biopsy and had four children, aged between two and eleven, who she missed terribly. The sad thing was that they never once came to visit her.

My struggle was with Sharon's negativity. She never had anything positive to say and she complained about everything, from the side-effects of the drugs to the staff. I did feel desperately sorry for her, but at times wanted to shake her and tell her to get on with it.

Sharon reminded me of Cathy, the woman I'd known at the RNZN hospital. Cathy had small children, but never got to see them. She spent a year in the hospital, never had visitors in all of that time, and died in the hospital two years later. Alone.

Sharon finished her cigarette and I wheeled her back to the ward. "Take care," I said. "Let me know how you get on."

2 November, 2000 (Thursday)

Sharon got her results today. I saw her in the coffee shop that afternoon being wheeled around by her husband. She was crying and I couldn't see her children. I wanted to give her a hug.

I was booked in for a post-op CT scan in the morning. I had not had a CT scan before and looked at the machine curiously. It wasn't a cocoon like the MRI, just a concave half-ring. I sat on the table and waited for the nurse.

The professor popped in during his evening rounds, accompanied by Michael, the registrar. "Results tomorrow!" he bellowed.

Due to the local anaesthetic, my forehead had swollen and the swelling was slowly moving around my face. It was a strange feeling, and I queried it with the prof. "Quite normal," he said, and with that moved on to the next room.

3 November, 2000 (Friday)

The big day. Deep down, I knew what the verdict was going to be – the biopsy was merely a clarification process. But always the optimist, I prayed for the 2%.

More important to me was the opportunity to talk to the professor about my future and treatments. He began with, "You have an anaplastic astrocytoma Grade 3 with an area turning to Grade 4… You're very young to have this type of tumour."

I had no emotion; it was no surprise to me really. Collectively we had made a list of questions to pose to the professor, so I began working through the list.

Questions for the Prof!

- What should the first stage of treatment be, in your opinion?
- When should the treatment start?
- When do the stitches come out?
- Are the suspect areas malignant? Can these be zapped with stereotactic radiotherapy?
- Is it operable/part-operable?
- Chemotablets. What are the side effects? Effect on life? How long?
- How will my flying career be affected?
- What resources are available over the course of treatment?
- Right to benefits?
- Affect on driver's licence?

Mum then spoke. "I'm going home on the 13th of November… Does Cam need help while being treated?"

I scoffed quietly, while the professor came to my rescue by saying, "Madam, he is not sick."

Dad continued with the questions.

- Steroids? How long does Cam take them for? Any swelling after steroids have stopped? Side effects coming off them?
- When should the next MRI scan be taken? How often will

one be done?
- When can Cam wash his hair?
- When should Cam meet with Professor Whittle next?
- Should we be reading information concerning Cam's tumour?
- Is stress likely to cause seizures, and will they continue to occur only during sleep?
- How extensively should he exercise, and what kind?
- How important is regular sleep over this next period of recuperation?
- Effect of alcohol?
- Should I be treated in Edinburgh or Liverpool?

So many questions. It really was uncharted territory for us and we were going to need some help

I checked out after spending five days in hospital and we drove home to Edinburgh on the Saturday. I was worried about Sarah and the lectures she'd missed while caring for me. I was glad to be getting home for her sake.

Astrocytomas are the most common type of primary brain tumour. Most brain tumours are named after the cells from which they develop. Astrocytomas develop from star-shaped glial cells called astrocytes. They may occur anywhere in the central nervous system (CNS), including the brain, the brain stem, or the spinal cord. Treatment usually includes surgery, radiation therapy and sometimes chemotherapy.

Anaplasia is the term used to describe the characteristic pattern in which tumour cells grow without form, structure or orientation to one another. An astrocytoma is assigned a grade according to its degree of anaplasia. Tumours are graded 1 to 4. Grade 1 and 2 tumors are slow-growing (benign). Grade 3 tumours will spread to surrounding brain tissue. Grade 4 astrocytomas, also known as glioblastoma multiform, grow quickly, spreading to other parts of the brain, and have the greatest degree of anaplasia and are therefore the most malignant (cancerous). How the astrocytoma is treated will depend on its grade. Grade 3-4 tumours respond well to radiotherapy, where as Grades 1-2 do not. Benign tumours may not be treated if they're not causing any deficiency. Best to leave well alone!

6 November, 2000

I started to think about the possibility of returning to flying. If the tumour shrank and I came off the anticonvulsant drug, Tegretol Retard, why couldn't I fly again? It made perfect sense.

I knew what I needed to do, and that was to take the offer of work from my boss and work in flight operations. It was important for me to stay in the aviation industry in some capacity. In whatever capacity!

That night, I searched the Internet for tumour websites and stumbled across a site for brain tumour survivors. I looked under the astrocytoma page and, to my delight, found about six names. But as I started to read their comments, I became increasingly horrified. The grammar and spelling was childlike, with the first three of the patients having obviously incurred some brain damage or having well-advanced tumours.

This was disappointing. I really needed to hear of someone who had had the same tumour as me and survived without any disability. I read on and there he was: Edward.

Edward was a fifty-six year-old married man with an eighteen year-old daughter. He was diagnosed with an anaplastic astrocytoma in 1979. As I read his story, my excitement grew. I e-mailed him straight away, told him my story and congratulated him. To know that someone had had exactly the same tumour as I and survived to live a long, full life did much for my determination. He became my hero. Ed gave me some advice on healthy living, but it was meditation that grabbed my interest. I did need to relax and meditation could well be the ticket. I noted in my diary, "Find out more about meditation!" I never did.

On the 8th of November, Mum left the United Kingdom and headed for home. The situation had become a financial strain on my parents, and the family business was suffering. I knew also that Mum missed her friends and their support. She'd seen for herself that I was okay, so she could leave in the knowledge that Dad would be here to see me through treatment – although both Dad and I would miss her terribly. We moved to a smaller rental property in Dalry.

13 November, 2000

I was awoken by Dad's footsteps. "Oh, shit!" I heard him say.

I was lying face down on the floor, having convulsed out of bed again. My excuse of rugby injuries weren't going to cover it this time... my grazes were much worse. How could I possibly fall out of a king-size bed? From that day on, I slept diagonally across the bed. How Sarah ever put up with this, I'll never know!

On the 13th of November I received a package and when I opened it a pile of cards spilled out. Unbeknown to me, my colleagues and friends had started a collection for me, and there were a number of cheques and well wishes from people – some of whom I had never met. I was deeply touched.

15 November, 2000

I met with Dr Gregor, the head of neuro-oncology. My treatment had now moved into her hands.

She greeted me with a warm smile and spoke with a German accent. It somehow reassured me, I think because of my fondness for Professor Warnke, who was also German. Dr Gregor had fiery red hair and spoke with an air of command and confidence, but at the same time there was a very sincere caring edge to her manner. I liked her immediately and she won my complete trust.

It had been suggested to me that my radiotherapy should begin immediately. However, Dr Gregor had come up with a new treatment plan. Initially, I was to commence treatment before Christmas, but this would have meant a gap in my radiation sessions between Christmas Day and New Year which would allow the tumour cells to regroup. A continuous period of radiation was preferred, so the decision was made to commence treatment in the New Year, starting on the 8th of January, 2001. During December my mask would be fitted and the trajectories of the radiation beams calculated.

I was pleased not to be starting therapy before Christmas – I'd still have hair! This was my first Christmas with Sarah and her family, and I wanted to feel normal.

Accompanying Dr Gregor was Shanne McNamara, a senior charge

nurse in the oncology department. Shanne was a trained nurse but her job was to look after patient welfare, which I'm sure she did well beyond that which her job description demanded of her. Once Dr Gregor had finished, Shanne and the charge nurse pounced, asking if there was anything I needed. Did I have enough medication, steroids? What were my travel arrangements? Did I need financial support? They couldn't have been more helpful.

22 November, 2000

As I stood over the sink doing dishes, I felt a rush of blood through my body. I could hear my head pulsating with my heartbeat. It was like nothing I'd ever experienced before.

"Whoaaaa!" I started to move towards my room, but a wave of nausea came over me so I crouched down, then felt dizzy so I lay down. I smelt a strong smell like ammonia, but there was nothing there. My palms were sweating and it was as though I was dreaming but I was still awake. Like a strange sense of déjà vu.

I felt scared. Dad crouched down over me and comforted me.

29 November, 2000

I saw a beggar in the street, a common enough sight for Edinburgh. Usually I was sympathetic, but this particular guy annoyed me. His sign read "Homeless and hopeless". I thought how lucky he was – after all, he had his health. I almost went up and told him so, but bit my tongue and continued to walk.

26 November, 2000

My friend Gareth rang, relating a telephone conversation he'd had with Paul. Paul had told him of my good result from the "autopsy", to which Gareth had responded, "I've never heard of anyone's hearing his own *autopsy* result!"

I laughed.

30 November, 2000

I had an appointment with my GP, Dr Laird, to collect my Tegretol Retard pills, an anticonvulsant medication. I enjoyed collecting my medication in person, because it afforded a chat with Dr Laird, which was always worthwhile.

While waiting for my prescription, I asked if I could read my file, and I started flicking through the notes. There were countless letters to and from Dr Laird, Professor Whittle, Dr Mumford, and insurance companies.

Then something caught my eye: a letter from Dr Gregor addressed specifically to Dr Laird that had not been intended for my eyes. Scanning the letter, I read: "Given Cameron's age, fitness and attitude, I see long-term remission of this tumour as a reality."

My eyes filled with tears. This was my first material glimmer of hope. Not words spoken to me to perk me up, but real, hard evidence. I was overjoyed. It felt like I'd been given a new zest for life.

9 December, 2000

Working at my computer, I was suddenly overcome by a wave of nausea. I felt dizzy, then had that same strange dream. I felt scared, although the episode only lasted a few minutes. I tried to make sense of it all. I'd had that dream before, but for the life of me couldn't remember it.

What was happening to me? Why?

I went back to the computer and searched the Internet under "seizures". To my amazement I found out exactly what I was looking for – my symptoms outlined almost word for word.

Extract taken from the British Epilepsy Association.

The Temporal Lobe

If a simple seizure originates in the temporal lobe, quite a wide variety of symptoms can occur. This is because the functions of the temporal lobe are quite varied. As with all types of epilepsy, each person is different and straightforward comparisons are not always possible.

Usually, someone having a simple partial seizure originating in the temporal lobe will experience an intense feeling, for example, sudden fear or happiness. They may have an extremely vivid memory flashback or strong sense of déja vu. Unpleasant smells or tastes and an unpleasant sensation in the stomach are also possible symptoms.

These symptoms are often called an "aura" and can act as a warning for people with complex partial seizures. During simple partial seizures, the person remains fully conscious and the seizure is usually very brief. Often it is only the intensity and suddenness of these feelings that differentiates between someone having a usual déja vu experience, for example, and someone having a simple partial seizure.

9 December, 2000

It was Saturday night. Sarah and I headed into the city to enjoy the Edinburgh nightlife.

A temporary ice-skating rink had been set up in Princess Street Gardens, and Sarah dragged me down to have a go. As we skated, I watched the snow fall and the glistening ice forming on whatever it touched. I felt the cold on my face and watched the warm breath exhaling from our mouths. The colours of Christmas were everywhere, and the laughter of children rang out. The sky was clear and the stars shone brightly, forming a magical canopy above us.

I watched Sarah intently as she skated, the sparkle in her eyes, her smile. I felt so in love and so alive…

***

By late December the work on my flat was finished and we were able to move in, much to our relief.

The day before my treatment began, I was excited: excited about finally getting treatment for my tumour, and being on the way to getting well. I had faith in and respect for the doctors I'd met. I had no doubt that what I was doing was the best thing for me.

My diary entry read: "The fight begins!"

8 January, 2001 (Monday)

Dad drove me to the hospital, cursing everyone on the road but himself as he did so. I'd come to ignore this ritual of his.

I jumped out and walked to the oncology department, inhaling the fresh morning air with confidence. "The fight begins," I smirked to myself.

Just before the session, I was met by one of the senior radiographers. She was a warm, middle-aged woman who asked me if I was all right. Did I want to ask anything? "No, let's rock on!" I replied, thrusting my left fist in the air.

"Okay, let's rock on!" she mimicked me in her crisp English accent, bringing a smile to my face.

I lay down on the bench on my back, and a mask was fitted. Memories of claustrophobia flooded back and I prayed that I wouldn't have a fit. But it was quick: three shots of radiation and ten minutes later I was finished.

No worries there, I reflected, walking back to the car. Dad had found a car park – albeit illegal – which made me smile.

I was told to expect some tiredness towards the end of the day, and sure enough, I did. As the treatment progressed, I could sense something was going on in my head. It was as if a reaction to the radiation was taking place. Something had been stirred up in my brain – and it didn't like it.

This poem was written by a young girl who died of cancer. She was just eleven years old.

Slow Dance

Have you ever watched kids?
On a merry-go-round?

Or listened to the rain
Slapping on the ground?
Ever followed a butterfly's erratic flight?
Or gazed at the sun into the fading night?
You better slow down.
Don't dance so fast.
Time is short.
The music won't last.

Do you run through each day
On the fly?
When you ask, "How are you?"
Do you hear the reply?
When the day is done
Do you lie in your bed
With the next hundred chores
Running through your head?
You'd better slow down
Don't dance so fast.
Time is short.
The music won't last.

Ever told your child,
We'll do it tomorrow?
And in your haste,
Not see his sorrow?
Ever lost touch,
Let a good friendship die
'Cause you never had time
To call and say "Hi"?
You'd better slow down.
Don't dance so fast.
Time is short.
The music won't last.

When you run so fast to get somewhere
You miss half the fun of getting there.
When you worry and hurry through your day,
It is like an unopened gift...
Thrown away.
Life is not a race.
Do take it slower
Hear the music
Before the song is over.

***

I learnt I was to meet with the oncologist every Wednesday at 10.00am.
This became an appointment I was to enjoy.

10 January, 2001

Max greeted me; a young registrar with short-cropped hair and a
beaming smile. We're going to hit it off, I thought.

He was accompanied by two nurses and a social worker, eager to
support me. Max gave me an overview of the treatment and showed
me the size of the area being treated. It was bigger than I'd realised –
twelve by twelve centimetres from the side, and nine by nine centimetres at the front, therefore covering a large part of my brain. At least
they'll get it all, I thought.

As I left, the nurse asked me if I had enough drugs. Steroids?
"Oh, I'm not on steroids," I replied, "but I'll have some anabolic
ones!" Max laughed and I gave him a high five on the way out.

13 January, 2001

My first tonic-clonic seizure for about five weeks came on a Saturday
morning, almost on cue. Sarah had stayed over and it was nice to have
her there for support. During the fit, my toenails scratched some paint
off my newly painted wall. This pissed me off, and hurt!

As the weekend drew to a close, I thought how nice it was to feel normal over the few days that I didn't have therapy. It was a time for my body to recover, and I hadn't felt tired in the late afternoon as I would do during the week, when I was getting treated.

15 January, 2001

After coming home from therapy, I felt nauseous. I hadn't felt sick before. I lay down on the wooden floor and reached for a bucket, which I promptly vomited into.

Feeling better, I stood up and prepared another wall for painting. Dad had been hard at work and my episode had gone unnoticed. I grabbed at my hair to see if the moulting had started, but nothing. I continued this daily ritual until, on the 24th of January, three hairs fell out. Talk about an anticlimax!

But by Monday, the 29th of January, all the hair that had come into contact with the radiation had fallen out. This left me with a patchy head of hair. It made me look sick, and I hated it. It was a constant reminder of my illness.

31 January, 2001

I wondered if the cancer could spread to other parts of my body. I mentioned my concern to Sarah. It had worried her too, and she had already researched the possibility. "It won't spread," she said.

I also worried about the effect on my motor skills, but I tended to keep my concerns about the tumour's side-effects to myself.

1 February, 2001

My libido had been gradually dropping, and now I couldn't even manage an erection. Most red-blooded males have something of a degree in masturbation, but for me it had become a fruitless exercise. I'd been expecting this temporary lack of sexual function, but it came as a shock all the same.

4 February, 2001

I had my first simple partial seizure for six weeks. Nothing appeared to provoke it, but nothing could prepare me for what I was about to experience in the coming week. I documented my seizures in the hope of finding some pattern. They occurred like clockwork, almost to the minute.

Mon 5 Feb	Tues 6 Feb	Wed 7 Feb	Thurs 8 Feb	Fri 9 Feb
-	-	0700	0700	-
-	-	1330	1300	1230
-	1600	-	1550	-
1800	1800	1730	-	-
-	2015	2015	2000	-
2330	2230	2230	-	-
-	0001	0130	-	-

Late afternoon on Tuesday the 6th, I was walking into town when my left leg suddenly gave way. I collapsed onto the pavement, knowing what was happening but unable to interrupt the flow of the seizure. The smells and strange thoughts began to take over. Still very conscious, I crawled to the steps of a nearby building and sat down.

The seizure passed and I thought about why I'd collapsed. I remembered that the right hemisphere of the brain controls the left side of the body. Ahh... that's why only my left leg was affected.

7 February, 2001

As I experienced the multiple simple partial seizures, I tried to understand the strange recurring dream and overwhelming fear that came with them. I described it in my diary as feeling that I was about to die in the next five minutes.

It was a terrible feeling of solitude and impending death. I needed to see an oncologist, and arranged an appointment for the next day.

8 February, 2001

My anticonvulsant medication was increased by 100mg, and I noticed an immediate effect. The following day the seizures dropped to just one.

11 February, 2001

Random childhood memories flooded my head. They were so obscure, but they were a nice experience. So many good memories. I wondered if my brain was trying to offload information. Spring cleaning, perhaps?

13 February, 2001

Peter Symes, a close family friend, died after a battle with bowel cancer. I was sad, but it made me realise that I wasn't alone.
I wondered how cancer patients died. Do they know? Are they in pain? I felt for his son, Wymond, who had been a close schoolmate. I needed to call him, but even in my situation I still couldn't think of what I could say.

14 February, 2001

"Watch out for the sun," Max advised me at our weekly appointment. "You're vulnerable, having had the radiotherapy."
I laughed – "Sun in the UK!?" – then nodded to show my understanding.

16 February, 2001

My last day of treatment! It was a beautiful, crisp, frosty morning covered with brilliant blue sky. I felt fantastic.
I met most of the doctors and oncology nurses that had treated me over the past three months. They all commented on my attitude, and how positive I'd been. It felt good, and I was humbled by their interest in me.

18 February, 2001

Andrew Schache, a friend from New Zealand, e-mailed me to say his cancer had spread to his brain. The e-mail was riddled with mistakes, which concerned me. I wrote back immediately and we discussed our cancers and how we would fight them.

28 February, 2001

Dad flew out today and as he walked through the departure gate I saw him for the man he was: an extremely gentle and loving person, devoted to his family. He had spent six months toiling for me, but never once uttered a word of complaint. He'd put months of work into the flat, and had suffered personally and financially.

He didn't expect a thank you. He did it all for me, and all he wanted in return was to receive the love of his son. I cried. I had given him a hug, but had forgotten to tell him I loved him. I wished I had. At that moment I was a little boy again, needing his dad. A father had found his son again - I just hoped he knew it.

"It is not flesh and blood, but the Heart, which makes us fathers and sons."

Friedrich von Schiller

Andrew Schache died today. I was stunned. I had talked with him just a few days ago and we had made a pact to beat our cancers together. This was too close to home. I couldn't understand, or make any sense of it.

2 March, 2001

I missed Dad and our little routines. The house seemed very empty without him. It was as much his home as mine. There were reminders of him everywhere. I became quite homesick and made a call to staff travel. Within a matter of hours, I was on my way home.

5 March, 2001

I sat in economy, the prospect of a twenty-four hour flight ahead of me. I reflected on the excitement of my flight to the United Kingdom some three years before, and the anticipation of a new career, a new life and all the adventures that lay ahead. Who'd have known? I couldn't help but feel sad.

It's not what you get, it's the way you deal with it that's important. – Auntie Anne

26 March, 2001

I returned to Scotland, refreshed after three weeks of beaches, beers and barbecues.

27 March, 2001

My hair had started growing back slowly, so I decided to continue cutting it short. I was in Forfar, visiting Sarah's parents, and paid a visit to the local barber. Explaining to him what had happened to my hair, I asked for a number one all over. Before I could stop him, he'd vigorously removed all my side! What!? They'd taken some time to grow, and when I wore a bandanna I looked normal.

"And your eyebrows, sir?" he asked.

I gasped in horror. "I'm quite fond of my eyebrows, thanks!" I paid him quickly and left.

1 April, 2001

I started to become aware of an odd phenomenon as I drifted off to sleep. I'd see a flash of light, like the release of an electrical charge. It would burn onto my retina like a camera flash and startle me. I always thought it was an impending seizure, but there was never any correlation.

21 April, 2001

More random memories. This time, they covered the last ten to fifteen years, not childhood as before. I wondered if it was because my mind was idle and looking for additional stimulation.

1 May, 2001

I returned to work as a ground instructor at the invitation of my boss Captain Bill Hanton. I was suspended from flying duties pending the outcome of a medical review with the Civil Aviation Authority. Bill's support during my illness was remarkable, and knowing that my position with the company was safe was a breastplate in the armour that I used to fight my cancer.

8 June, 2001

I awoke to find Sarah crying. I cuddled her and asked her what was wrong.

"I'm worried about the future. I wish I knew that you were going to be okay... it scares me, Cam."

I'd been waiting for this, and was surprised it had taken this long. Sarah had been studying medicine at university and had been doing neurology that week. There had been a lecture about brain tumours that day. She didn't attend.

I whispered in her ear, "You need to board my train. Have you got your ticket?"

I smiled, and out of her tears she said, "Yep!"

"I need to have you on my train, Honey," I told her. "I'm going to beat this thing and I need to have you aboard."

She smiled, I hugged her, and we fell asleep.

29 June, 2001

Although my new hair was growing much slower than my old hair, it was time for another haircut. It was time to cultivate my old "big hair".

With memories of my last disastrous visit to a barber fresh in my mind, I went to my local barber in Edinburgh. I was very specific and I asked for a flat top. She did a wonderful job and I could see my old self coming back in the mirror.

I emerged from the salon delighted, and strutted down the street like a bad Elvis impersonator. For the first time in three months, I was in public without a hat or bandanna, and it felt great!

I used to have a saying: "If you look good, you feel good, and if you feel good, you can do anything." It summed up perfectly how I felt that day. I was so excited that I rang Mum. My confidence had returned.

10 July, 2001

I was back working in Aberdeen and Sarah rang to give me the date of my final scan. It was going to be a CT scan on the 1st of August – only three weeks away! I had butterflies in my stomach. I'd waited a long time for this day. It was all I could think about and it occupied my thoughts over the weeks to come.

I dreamt of coming home to a party with all my friends, having had the good news of total remission. Was my dream going to come true? I couldn't help but think about the enormity of this day. It would determine if I was going to live or die.

I had to regroup and take control, before these thoughts consumed me. Hilton was coming up, which was just as well as I was going to need my friends. The next three weeks would be tough, but I couldn't deny the mounting excitement.

12 July, 2001

My childhood flashbacks continued and became more frequent. The memories tended to focus around my family and my earliest years. I thought about the healing process, and I could see the need to return to some form of study to help my brain heal.

15 July, 2001

I contemplated death and tried to understand what it would be like. It can't be that bad; plenty of people have died before me – I wasn't going to be the first. What would happen to my soul? Would it eternally wander the world in some sort of dream state? Will I see my niece grow up? Will I meet my deceased grandparents?

Although not particularly spiritual, I believed in God. I took comfort in the knowledge that death would be a peaceful experience, and it no longer scared me.

26 July, 2001

The 1st August scan had consumed me for a month. The future of my life and flying career weighed heavily. But I was excited, and was going to greet the day with as much optimism as possible.

I was also feeling good. I'd had just one seizure since the end of treatment, and it was an indication to me that my brain was healing. I tried exercising, but feared this would cause a seizure, so rested while keeping my brain active. I firmly believed that learning new things, and processing new information, was the key to the healing process. I was prepared for bad news if it came, but my focus was on the tumour having gone into total remission, leaving only scar tissue behind. I figured it was this scar tissue that was responsible for the simple partial seizures.

1st August, 2001

The day of my scan. When it was over I e-mailed my family and friends.

The email read:

My scan was at 1.30pm on the 1st of August and took just ten minutes. I had eighty minutes to wait around for the results. Two friends from school who were working in London, Hilton and Chris, came up to be with me for a bit of moral support.

Ten minutes before my consultation, a woman came into the

waiting room and told me they wanted to run through some tests – co-ordination, memory and motor skills tests. I freaked (internally that is; no, I didn't run around the room in tears, waving my arms). All I could think of was that they had found something bad, maybe my tumour had grown and the tests were to see how demented I was becoming. I gave both the guys high fives and went off to the exam room. I "smoked" the tests and said to the woman, "So is this standard for all patients?" "Oh yes," she replied, so I gathered my heart off the floor and pondered why she hadn't told me that in the first place.

I was called into the consultation room at 3.00pm Dr Niblock met me; she was about my age. She had a warm beaming smile, and as we sat down, she said, "You're going to be okay!"

There was a silence as those words resonated around the room, and the enormity of what they meant sunk in. Tears welled up in my eyes and I could hear Sarah crying. She continued, "The tumour has shrunk and what remains is static and will go away over time. Some scar tissue will remain. How have you been?"

I choked; I struggled with the words and fought tears of relief and joy as I described my wellbeing over the last few months. I glanced over at the guys, who both had a tear in their eye. I was emotionally drained and I gave her a hug. "Thank you," I said.

She showed me the scans and the comparison with my original scan back in July last year. Seeing the difference gave me the final inner peace I had been waiting for.

She had said that many of the nurses and doctors that I had dealt with had all been sneaking a look at the result, which was nice. I had made many friends at the hospital.

Consultation over, I walked outside, thrust my fists in the air, had a group hug, and vowed I would start going to church to make up for all the prayers I had made over the last year.

From being told a year ago, that I had five years to live and that they would try to prolong my life and give me a few good years, to being well again, and being told to go away and enjoy my life, was just an emotional high of epic proportion for me, and I promptly went off and got drunk!

That evening Sarah, Chris, Hilton and I went into town to celebrate. I was in a world of my own, on a natural euphoric high. As we walked into the first bar, *Pride* by U2 was thundering out of the speakers. It was like being hit by a bolt of lightning. All afternoon I had wanted to shout out loud my sheer joy, and by now I was ready to explode. On hearing that song I leapt onto the podium and danced like I had never danced before. The club was packed with people but I didn't care; I didn't even notice. That night was mine and I was going to live like there was no tomorrow.

2 August, 2001

I went to the local supermarket and, on the way home, three boys aged about seven or eight approached me. The lad on the right asked me if I'd like to buy a postcard or programme. Apparently the boys had picked these up from the local movie theatre for free, and I smiled. I admired their initiative, and they reminded me of myself at their age.

Seeing they were about to lose a quick sale, the middle boy said, "Half the money goes to cancer research."

"Does it?" I enquired, "Do you boys know how important cancer research is?"

I got an unconvincing reply, but emptied the coins from my wallet. Looking towards the middle boy, I said, "You may have a pound. That's fifty pence for you and fifty pence for cancer research."

I turned to the lad to my left, who'd had nothing, and said, "Here's fifty pence for you too. That's to make sure your friend here gives his to cancer research."

He held out his hand to shake on it. "It's a deal!" I gave him a sly wink and chuckled as I walked away.

Drifting off to sleep that night, I pictured a white ball. It was the size of a golf ball and as white and smooth as porcelain. It represented what was left of my tumour. Gone was any sign of black – the cancer. It was pure white. Over the following months the ball in my dream would get smaller and smaller, and move further and further away from me.

4 August, 2001

I opened my e-mail inbox to find an e-mail from Mum. Mum's e-mail read:

> Once upon a time there was a little boy who loved to play with toy guns. Many a battle was waged with the neighbourhood children. He was the Captain; they were his men. Battles were fought and won. He was always the Hero. Eventually, the children grew up and moved away, each to his own career, but this little boy never stopped wanting to be a Hero. He joined the Navy but there were no wars. He became a pilot – he was in command, in control, but there was no war to win, no battle to be waged. Until one day, without warning, he found himself in the midst of a battle terrible and frightening. The enemy came at night while he slept. "That's not fair," he cried. "Where are my soldiers? I can't fight this by myself." Then he looked within himself and found an army so strong nothing could stand in its way. The enemy was vanquished; he had won his battle. He is the greatest Hero of them all.

> Love,
> Mum

8 August, 2001

I sent a card to Dr Gregor to thank her and the team for all they had done for me. I have tremendous respect for her and the many nurses, doctors and physicians who treated me. They are all a credit to their profession and I wanted to show my gratitude.

10 August, 2001

I arranged to meet with children from the Maggie Centre. This was a unit set up for young people with cancer, and I was looking forward to the meeting immensely.

I pondered my reason for organising an activity with them in the first place. Who was I doing this for? Them? Me? Or both? I was desperate to give something back in return for the treatment that I had received. After my parents' experience with that awful woman from the support group, I wanted to be a positive role model and give the kids hope. At seventeen, your life is just starting, you're thinking about your career, you have dreams and desires. I wanted to be someone they could look at and think: "He survived, so can I. He's an airline pilot! I can be anything I want to!"

14 August, 2001

Sarah and I arrived early at the Maggie Centre, not really knowing what to expect, or what was expected of me. I just hoped to get a chance to tell my story.

Andrew met us and showed us around. The Centre is an old renovated stable. It looked like a child's bedroom, with toys strewn around the place, books, bright colours everywhere. It was perfect.

Andrew was a nurse but employed to look after the Maggie Centre. He was young and had a bubbly personality – ideally suited to his role. I studied him closely, remembering my parents' unpleasant experience with the brain tumour support group.

I looked forward to meeting the kids, and they began to arrive in dribs and drabs. There were six in total, as well as a social worker called Hans. He was a grafter, the sort of guy who'd bend over backwards for you, and then ask what else he could do.

Invited to talk, I began my story. My main focus was the importance of staying positive, and the need to control your illness and not let your illness control you.

As I talked, I could see a boy called Jamie becoming increasingly agitated. He was twenty-two years old and had throat cancer. He'd already had an operation and undergone both chemo and radiotherapy.

I paused and he suddenly spoke. "So you've been given a 100% recovery prognosis?"

"Yes," I replied.

"Well, I've been just as positive, and I've been given six to twelve months to live!"

He stared at me. I could see in his eyes that he was angry, and was

45

venting his anger and frustration at me. I didn't know what to say.

Andrew picked up the conversation and talked in support of what I had said. I began talking again and we had a group discussion on what doctors should tell patients about the prognosis. I mentioned how Professor Whittle was able to lift the spirits of my family by being so positive, and that, in turn, this positivity was the impetus for the way I'd dealt with my tumour.

Jamie wasn't convinced. "So you think they should lie?" he said. "I wanted to know the truth."

"No," Andrew and I replied simultaneously, "not lie. Just turn it a little. They can give hope, and hope can lead to self-healing."

Jamie was a strong young man, there was no denying it, and I admired his bravery. I wanted to continue the conversation with him one-on-one, and would get that chance when he came flying with me.

25 August, 2001

Before departure, I took Jamie to the business class lounge. I'd arranged to have at least forty-five minutes to talk before the flight. As we walked in, the receptionist reminded me that I wasn't allowed in the lounge in uniform. I asked Jamie to wait outside and pulled out the "kids with cancer" story. That saw the end of her interruption.

As Jamie spoke to me, I thought about what the impact would have been on me had I known about my tumour at his age. I wouldn't have been able to join the Navy and I certainly wouldn't have had a flying career. Here was a courageous young man who had just as many dreams as I or anyone else, but he'd been cut off at the knees. I was deeply moved by Jamie's plight. He's going to have fun today, I thought. I'll make sure of it!

Jamie got to ride in the cockpit on both sectors of the flight, from Edinburgh down to Manchester and back. He absolutely adored it, and it made me feel good to do something for someone who had been through as much as he had. The attention I gave Jamie meant a great deal to him, which he expressed in a letter to me afterwards.

Two years on, Jamie made a full recovery. There is no doubt that he beat his cancer through his own strength of character. He has moved into his own apartment and has returned to Edinburgh University to complete his accountancy degree.

*****

But what next for me? I had now given something back, and although I'd continue to try to put something back where I could, I was also ready to put the whole tumour saga behind me. I felt closure. It was time to get on with my life.

There were many positives that had come out of my illness, probably the biggest being the reconnection I'd made with my parents. I had also changed. I was less agitated, more thoughtful and self-aware. In understanding myself better, I also saw the positive and negative impact I had the potential to have on those close to me. I knew why my first marriage had failed. I knew how to make my next marriage work.

27 August, 2001

I'd been corresponding with June, a woman whose son had a brain tumour. She was looking for reassurance, which I could relate to, having watched my own mother.

June told me her son had a pilocytic astrocytoma tumour, located in the left parietal lobe, so I searched the Internet to find out where in the brain the parietal lobe was. While searching, I came across the functions of the temporal lobe – where my tumour had been. As I read what functions may or may not be affected, I was intrigued. It made a lot of sense. Here were many of the behavioural and physiological effects that I had experienced over the last eighteen months.

Areas impacted by the temporal lobe included auditory memories (related to hearing) and some hearing; visual memories and some vision pathways; other memory; music; fear; as well as some language, speech and behaviour.

What really attracted my attention was the mention of fear, other memories and the area of language and speech. Pieces of a puzzle suddenly fell into place for me. Fear had characterised my simple partial seizures, but I'd also noticed how I often startled easily now, or suffered anxiety without apparent reason. Although my long-term memory was fine, at times I had difficulty recalling information from my short-term memory. And my speech and language had definitely been impacted in some way, as I often mispronounced words.

Few and far between as they mostly were, these side-effects were very noticeable to me. Understanding why I had them helped. My tumour had been irradiated, but the remaining scar tissue could well cause such function deficiency.

4 September, 2001

I began to take on more responsibility at work, something I desperately needed. I wanted a challenge; I wanted to feel I was moving on with life. It was also important to feel I was contributing on the same level as the others in the training team.

I began running the refresher courses, designed to give existing company line pilots a revision of aircraft systems. I enjoyed these immensely and it gave me a chance to get out of the office and travel around Britain.

10 November, 2001

I felt I had reached normality in my life. My brain tumour was virtually a memory, the daily ritual of drug-taking being my only reminder.

But things aren't always so simple, and at a party on the 9th of November, I noticed a deficiency in my short-term memory. I struggled to recall names, dates and basic words that would normally have come to me easily. It alarmed me. The number of occurrences was almost overwhelming, and it was embarrassing as I struggled to speak with people after long pauses of thought. Over the past few months, I'd had a few problems recalling details, but suddenly I was involved in numerous conversations and the deficiency in my short-term memory was all too evident. I hoped that maybe I was overreacting. Time would tell.

15 November, 2001

An opportunity arose for me to go to Paris and do the Embraer 145 Simulator course. I took it up with gusto. The opportunity to fly a new aeroplane – a jet no less, even if it was a simulator – was too good to pass by. I was flying again, if only for a short while. It was heaven.

19 November, 2001

I'd felt a little faint all day, that pre-seizure feeling I'd come to know all too well. Having had a simple partial seizure the night before, I decided to have an early night.

As I lay in bed, out of the blue, the song, *I Don't Believe in If Anymore* by Roger Whittaker rang through my head. It was so clear and so real that I was stunned. Roger Whittaker was a folk singer of the 1970s, whose album my father played when I was a child. I'd not heard this song for at least twenty-five years. This was the clearest of all my random childhood memories, and it comforted me. It was a special and distinctive reminder of my father.

I read recently that it is a common defence mechanism of our psyche to revert to childhood memories during times of stress and anxiety. Pre-adolescence for most of us is a time of security and happiness.

3 December, 2001

Apart from Sarah, hanging on to the hope that one day I would return to flying had kept me sane throughout this upheaval in my life. I knew it was going to be a battle to return to flying and maybe a fruitless one, but I'd overcome so much already that I began to believe it was possible. If at any stage I felt that I would be a danger to the passengers and crew I would not have pursued the issue. But I felt fine and saw no reason why I shouldn't pilot a commercial aeroplane.

The medical division of the Civil Aviation Authority had appeared to many pilots to be an organisation that, although very black and white in its approach, was also on our side. If you had been working for an airline, it was far more likely that the CAA would take a softer approach when reviewing your condition and ability to return to flying.

So my expectation was that I'd serve a period of time on the ground while I proved to the CAA that I had not developed a seizure condition – perhaps three years, while I came off the medication.

Fellow pilots who'd been through similar plights advised me through the Internet that investigations were usually drawn-out affairs. It was important to my case to find a consultant who was prepared to tell the CAA what they wanted to hear.

Dr Colin Mumford was the obvious choice for me, so I asked Colin to approach the CAA on my behalf. I expected a meeting with Colin to talk about my course of action and how I would structure my case. I'd been gathering a lot of information, including examples of pilots with various neurological conditions that had returned to flying, albeit on a two-pilot restriction.

5 December, 2001

The position of Security Manager had become vacant at work, and I'd been advised by the Flight Operations Director to apply. The role had become high profile following September 11, and it offered me a chance to cement my place in the company. As a requirement, I would need to attend courses in London and Manchester. I was chosen for the position and it did much to help me overcome the loss of my flying.

6 December, 2001

I noted in my diary, "When life seems to deal you constant misfortune, it just gets better!"

10 December, 2001

Sarah and I flew out to New Zealand. I wanted to show her where I had come from and what made me who I am. I also wanted to give her the time of her life, and, of course, show her off to everyone!

12 January, 2002

When I arrived back from New Zealand, the first piece of mail I opened was from the CAA. Why they'd written to me at this stage, I wasn't sure, but I opened it nonetheless. The letter read:

We have recently received a detailed report from Dr Colin Mumford regarding your astrocytoma. I have discussed your case with our consultant advisor in neurology here at Aviation House. I regret that although you have no significant neurological deficit, the fact that you are taking long-term anticonvulsants and have an unacceptably high risk of seizure in the future means that I will have to assess you as "long-term unfit" for all classes of JAA medical certification.

I stared blankly at the letter, disbelieving. What was this, "no significant" business? I had *no* neurological deficit! And as for being a long-term drug dependant, I'd been told that I could come off the drugs whenever I wanted to! I also hadn't had a tonic-clonic in over a year!

I was angry because I'd been told that my flying career was basically over, and even more so, I'd been told through a letter it was over because there was a big "what if?" around my future. This was bullshit! They were telling me I couldn't get a licence because I might have a seizure. I'd flown with pilots who were far more likely to have a heart attack while flying than I was to suffer a seizure!

I couldn't help but wonder what exactly Colin had said, and if he'd somehow sold me out. I had to see the head neurologist at Aviation House and put forward my case. I needed to voice my frustration and show this man, who had ended my career, that I was not just a number. I was a young man who was fit and well and had a passion for aviation. Five days later, I was on my way to Aviation House at Gatwick Airport.

1 February, 2002

I sat in the waiting room, looking around at the other pilots. Some were there for their first medical issue while others, like me, were awaiting decisions that could put an end to their careers.

Dr Merry called me in. Highly respected in his field, he was a distinguished man in his late fifties. He knew exactly why I was there, and immediately began talking to me about his decision.

When he apologised for notifying me by letter, I seized my opportunity and began to put my case forward. I began with the letter's unsubstantiated claims, moving on to the past cases that I had researched.

"I've spoken to guys who have had brain haemorrhages, strokes, operable brain tumours, and one chap who is prone to fainting, and fits when he faints," I explained. "They've all returned to flying. So why am I any different?"

"What it comes down to," Dr Merry said, "is the issue of the risk of a seizure. There is a 50% chance that your tumour will recur within five years, and a 75% chance that it will recur within ten years. This is an unacceptably high seizure risk."

"My frustration is that this is all based on 'what ifs'," I replied. "Could I, for example, return to flying if I were still in the clear after ten years?"

"No," he said. He sensed my frustration and leaned toward me as I continued to speak.

"Look, I'm a healthy young man," I said, "I've been flying since I was eleven years old – it's my life. Flying is everything to me."

I paused, and I could see that Dr Merry saw the pain in my eyes. "Hang in there old boy," he said.

I held out my hand and he shook it. "It's not over yet," I said with a smile.

"I admire your positivity, Cameron."

I thanked him for his time and left, knowing that at the very least, I'd struck a cord with Dr. Merry. It made me feel better to know that he knew who Cameron Fulljames was, and that I was a lot more than just the file number ATPL 338147A.

22 March, 2002

Following my consultation with Dr Merry, I pondered the realisation that I might never fly commercially again. Faced with the loss of my flying career – a job that was more like a hobby than a career – I realised I was going to have to look outside aviation for the first time to find my passion.

My life needed meaning and stimulation. If I were to stay in aviation, it would have to be in management, even though the thought of a desk job had always repulsed me. Flying was my lifeblood. The question was, with the end of flying, was it to be the death of me?

2 June, 2002

I organised a European holiday for Mum and Dad. It was important to me that they had a great time; I felt I owed it to them after all the stress and anguish they'd endured on their last visit when I was ill. The opportunity to spend quality time with them was equally important.

We had an amazing six weeks, covering Prague, Amsterdam, Scotland, Ireland and the Orkney Isles. It was trip I'll never forget.

16 July, 2002

I still thought about recurrence, just momentarily, every day. It wasn't a serious consideration, but it lingered in my subconscious.

18 July, 2002

Do we have a soul, or do souls live on in the memories of those we love?

I think we would all like to know that our lives would be remembered after we leave this earth. Kevin, my friend, died this morning after lying in an induced coma as a result of a car accident. My cousin Campbell's ex-wife Karen was also killed recently in a similar accident. I guess the longer you live, the more death you are exposed to.

But it hurts. Why do the good ones die and not the others? Is it just the law of averages? Or is God telling us that we are all vulnerable? I don't know. I wish I knew the answer.

"When you lose a person you love, you gain an angel you know."
Oprah Winfrey

22 July, 2002

I began giving advice to two guys who had had seizures, although neither were tumour-related. Both contacted me through a website for airline pilots.

It felt good to help young pilots, although I still felt angry about the verdict I'd received. It seemed so unfair. I couldn't help but feel that my case deserved more consideration and respect than it had been given.

4 August, 2002

Something happened one day at work that moved me deeply, and showed me how much the tumour had increased my awareness of other people.

Graeme, who recruited cabin crew, was laughing at an application from a woman who looked very simple in her application photo. "Imagine being faced with her in the aisle!" he laughed.

I looked at the photo and felt genuine sympathy for her, remembering my years of sending out applications to every airline in the United Kingdom, praying for a reply.

When he left the office, I rummaged through the rubbish and read her application, noting the obvious difficulty she had with writing and spelling.

The application read:

Working as cabin crew has been my main ambition since leaving primary school... Because I would like to make working as cabin crew a career this means that I would put in the maximum effort into my job prove to be capable, willing, and willing at all times.

My heart ached for her; I knew all too well the need for that first big break.

My CT scan was booked for the 4th of September. In the months leading up to it, I contemplated death. I felt death would be almost easy to deal with. It was as if I'd lived my life in the time span of thirty years, as opposed to the usual ninety-odd years.

Looking back, several factors had contributed to my experiencing a mild depression. Without flying, life seemed humdrum. Although busy in my personal life and job, I was in a rut , which I needed to do something about. Even my sex life continued to suffer, since my libido had maintained an almost non-existent level after radiotherapy. I was afraid I'd lose Sarah.

What neither Sarah nor I knew at this time was that there was a medical, as opposed to psychological, reason for my loss of sexual function. During treatment, the tumour was bombarded with radiation and my pituitary gland had been in the line of fire. The result was that my pituitary gland no longer functioned, causing my levels of testosterone and hydrocortisol to fall at an alarming rate.

Endocrinology pamphlet:

The pituitary gland, which is located in the centre of the skull, just behind the bridge of the nose, is about the size of a bean. It is an important link between the nervous system and the endocrine system and releases many hormones which affect growth, sexual development, metabolism and the system of reproduction.

1 September, 2002

Days before my scan, I tried to visualise the remains of my tumour. But there was nothing, only darkness.

4 September, 2002

Sarah came with me on the day of my scan. As we sat waiting, I remembered the day of my diagnosis and told Sarah about how I had received the prognosis, surrounded by medical students. Being told I had five years to live was still a vivid memory.

"They told you here!" Sarah exclaimed in disgust. "Yep," I replied.

My name was called and I leapt up, walking down the corridor as I'd done many times over the years. As I prepared to move into the scaner,

I tried again to visualise my tumour. There was still nothing. I chanted over and over, "Don't be there, don't be there," and clutched my Maori bone-carving necklace that symbolised mana (pride) and strength.

When it was over, we walked to the Department for Clinical Neurosciences to await the results. I had no real reason to doubt the outcome.

Dr Anna Gregor, the head of oncology, was scheduled to see me, and I was delighted. We'd become close over the years. Shanne McNamara was there as always, the heart and soul of the department.

I entered Dr Gregor's office. She smiled at me and announced, "The scans are good."

I looked at the X-rays with little emotion, my eyes drifting to other areas of my head. I looked with fascination at my eye sockets and ear canals which, when combined, looked like a cartoon face.

We started to talk about getting me back to flying, and Dr Gregor offered to submit a new report to the CAA. "That would be fantastic!" I exclaimed. My logic was: remove the tumour, remove the seizures, and there was no logical reason why I shouldn't return to flying!

I rang Mum as soon as I could. She was overwhelmed with joy. Having suffered terribly over the years of my illness, it was comforting to know this would be the end of her pain. I had vowed that, had my tumour showed signs of recurrence, I would not have told her until I had to. Mum said, "Ring your father - you don't know how much this will mean to him."

As I told people about the result, I used the analogy of an oil slick. My brain tumour was the oil slick which was killing wildlife (my healthy brain cells). My radiotherapy was the cleanup operation. On the 1st August, 2001, my CT scan had showed that the clean-up operation had been successful but there was still some oil along the beach (residual tumour and scar tissue). The scan on the 4th of September showed that the oil on the beach had now gone. There was still a risk of future oil slicks, but a risk I vowed never to contemplate again.

20 September, 2002

I thought about flying, and wondered, Will I ever accomplish my Everest?

22 September, 2002

It was time to come off my medication. I was still taking an average dose, so decided to drop to 100mg (half a tablet) every two weeks.

It started well, and I dropped the dose still further. I felt good and hoped my lack of libido would begin to return. At the end of the fourth week I stayed with Sarah's family in Forfar. We went out on Saturday night, and when we arrived home I was exhausted.

At 7.00am Sarah woke me – I'd had a seizure. I stood up and lost all control, urinating all over the floor. I felt drowsy, and drifted off to sleep again to the comfort of Sarah's voice. Four hours later, I felt somebody's arms around me. I could hear shouting, a commanding voice. It was Sarah's father, who was pulling my shoulders back onto the bed. I had had another seizure, but this time had fallen out of bed and cracked my forehead on the sofa bed. Blood was seeping from my left eye.

When I came to, I knew what had happened. The all-too-familiar signs of a tonic-clonic seizure were there: nausea, muscle and joint pain, and drowsiness.

Later that day I sat cupping my face in my hands, I looked up at Sarah and her mother and said, "I guess it's time to give up on the idea that I'll ever fly again."

14 October, 2002

I had made the decision to see a doctor (finally) to get my libido problem sorted. I booked into therapy, something I wasn't looking forward to. Sharing intimate details of my sex life with a stranger did not appeal.

Then my blood test results came back and I made an appointment with my GP to hear them. They'd obviously found something.

When I saw the GP and she showed me the results, a huge weight lifted off me. My testosterone levels had been tested, and while the normal range for an adult male was between ten and thirty, my level was one point nine! I joked that I was almost a woman! I was suffering from pituitary dysfunction, which meant I needed to see an endocrinologist.

My test results read:

Testosterone	1.9	(Normal 10–30)
Prolactin	756	(Normal 60–500)
Free T4	6	(Normal 8–27)
Normal TSH		

***

My endocrinologist was Professor Walker, who confirmed the low testosterone finding and queried the effect of radiotherapy on my pituitary gland. He prescribed hormone replacement therapy, including a monthly injection of Sustanon (testosterone) in the posterior and more drugs. Thankfully, the pile of pills was small; however, on top of my Tegretol, I would be taking hydrocortisone, Thyroxin and Sustanon for the rest of my life.

All this would have been easy to accept if I hadn't been told I was probably sterile as well. Because no one had suspected the impact on my pituitary gland, I had not been asked to supply a sperm sample for storage before my radiation treatment. I was a little angry that my inevitable sterility might have been avoided, but there was a glimmer of hope – a small window of opportunity to store good sperm before this function vanished without further drug treatment. I needed to do it immediately.

31 December, 2002

New Year's eve at 7.30 in the morning isn't the sexiest time of day; nevertheless, I made my way to the Reproductive Ward of the New Royal Infirmary.

I was suffering from embarrassment – as I was sure many other men had before me – as I handed my documents to the nurse at reception and was shown to my cubicle. It was plain and functional, with a small table and chair dominating the room. Next to them were a hand basin and toilet.

Looking about the room anxiously, my mind raced at the thought of trying to accomplish my mission without external stimulus. The nurse pointed to a grey box on the table, indicating that what I had been looking for was inside. Then she locked the door behind her, leaving me to use my body like an amusement park!

Armed with a receptacle two centimetres in diameter, several copies of *Whoppers* and *Big Ones* and with one foot jammed up against the door, I pulled off the task at hand!

***

On Friday, the 3rd January came the letter that held the fate of my flying career. It was written by the head of the Aeromedical Department of the CAA. The letter read:

> Dear Cameron,
> I sincerely regret that you have been assessed as "long-term unfit" to exercise the privileges of your pilot's licence in a private or professional capacity.
> I do appreciate that you feel well and I am glad this is the case, but the risk of future incapacitation exceeds that required for the issue of any form of medical certificate for flying.
> I have every sympathy with your situation, which I am aware you have had a lot of difficulty in accepting.
> I am very sorry that I am unable to return you to flying.
>
> With kind regards,
> Dr S. A. Evans

As I looked at the words, I desperately wanted to say, What about the others? It's not fair! But this time, it was time to let go.

February, 2003

It may have taken time, but I've at last made my peace with the reality that I'll never pilot a commercial aeroplane again.

I needed to put what had happened to me into perspective. I had beaten my cancer and become a better person for the experience. I was alive and a very lucky man! I had been reminded that there were so many more important things in life, and that love, family and friendships are the food for the soul.

There is a career out there for me that will fill the void, and I will love it! But from now on, I'll be "flying without wings!"

***

3 September, 2003
I had my final MRI scan; it was clear!

Less than two months after my final scan, I had developed partial paralysis down my left side. My eyesight was affected first. I began to have difficulties reading, and also my peripheral vision was poor. With a history of poor eyesight in the family, I was not concerned. I was thirty-three years old; after all, an age at which all of my family had received reading glasses.

11 October, 2003
While on a weekend away in Perthshire with Sarah, I had developed a prominent limp. My left leg had ceased to function properly. It felt "lazy." All I could do was swing it like a pendulum, supported by my right leg. As my leg gradually got worse in the coming weeks, my left arm began to feel the same way. Ever the optimist, I blamed this on hormones causing muscle weakness. Sarah disagreed and so I booked a consultation with Dr Anna Gregor.

18 October, 2003
As I walked back to my flat from Sarah's, I did so with extreme difficulty. I couldn't walk properly no matter how hard I concentrated. My eyes glazed over and I felt nauseous. I just had to get home. I felt as if my body were shutting down. When I finally got home, I collapsed onto the bed. I looked out through the open window at the sky and prayed to God for more time. I had too much to do, many things to

finish and I wasn't ready to go.

What was puzzling about the onset of what clearly was a rapid recurrence of my tumour was that I had suffered no headaches or seizures as a result.

29 October, 2003

"The boss is waiting for you," said Shaune. I smiled at her and walked into the DCN waiting room with Sarah. "What have you done?" enquired Dr Gregor. "Well, it's sort of why I have come to see you," I replied.

After some short tests, she said, "This is neurological, Cameron." She was disappointed. I could see it in her eyes and sensed it in her voice. She had experienced what Sarah later told me was a "heart sink," a medical professional term for a doctor's feeling of hurt and anguish towards their patient's prognosis.

It was going to be chemotherapy this time. I had had my quota of radiation. I just wanted to get started. I needed to throw my energy into a treatment plan and get my mind and body into the self-healing "groove." Chemo wasn't going to be easy; I knew that. But it was different this time. There was no "unknown" and I didn't have the loss of my career to think of.

3 November, 2003

I was scanned on the Monday, 3rd November. As I lay in the MRI, I listened to the music coming through the headphones. The lyrics of Annie Lennox reverberated around my head and I sang with her.

"Hey, hey, I saved the world today?

Everybody's happy now,

The bad thing's gone away."

As the word spread among my friends and colleagues, the offers of support flooded in: accommodation for my parents, transport for me to the hospital... My friends were rallying around me, and, oh, how I needed them. Day by day, as I waited for the pre-treatment consultation, I just got worse. Simple tasks like buttoning a shirt, tying shoelaces, eating with a knife and fork, became a nightmare and caused me huge frustration, which I tried to avoid. A kind word or message of encouragement by phone, card or by mouth went straight to my heart and gave me tremendous strength.

"Cam, you're one of the strongest people I know; you'll beat this bastard of a thing."

"If anyone can beat this, it's you, you're a fighter!"

5 November, 2003

As I waited in DCN to see Dr Gregor, a young couple sat beside me. The young woman was visibly upset, and it was apparent that she was about to receive a diagnosis. When I had finished reading my paper, I offered it to them. "Oh, we'll check our horoscopes, thank you," they said in unison. I smiled, remembering doing the same three years earlier. Needing to hear any form of confirmation and hope that you'll be okay, the horoscope can help, in a strange way. In August, 2000, mine read:

"You may be feeling apprehensive. Does Saturn's arrival in Gemini signify the start of a long saga of struggle? Not really. It's just that the next couple of years will have a recurring theme involving intermittent tests of your patience and your faith that will eventually leave you wiser and stronger in every sense. There will be many weeks, even months on end, when life is so joyous that you don't even notice it. This weekend though, you may get a taste of what the big challenge is all about."

The results of the scan were going to be merely a confirmation that my tumour had recurred. However, as before, the scan showed little. Dr Gregor could only say that is was likely that it had recurred deep within the brain region where scar tissue had remained after radiotherapy. Given the physical disabilities I was experiencing, recurrence was certain. "This is not life-threatening, but quick to return," she said, "and I would like to involve you in a clinical trial." I was very excited; an opportunity to help bring a new drug onto the market, and help others, was too good to miss.

The normal treatment for the recurrence of a high-grade glioma would be PCV (three chemotherapy drugs). The clinical trial was going to test the new drug Temodal against the old chemotherapy regime. I couldn't wait to start. I received confirmation the next day from Shaune that I would begin treatment on Wednesday the 12 th of November.

I had been randomised for PCV, the tried-and-tested chemotherapy, but I was disappointed not to be receiving the new, so-called wonder drug, Temodal. I was assured, however, that those on clinical trials always do better, because of the continuous monitoring. That was good enough for me! I needed to throw my energy into a treatment plan, to get my mind and body into the self-healing groove.

12 November, 2003

Dr. Sarah Erridge gave me a thorough explanation of the treatment plan and possible side-effects. PCV chemotherapy is administered as three different drugs:

- P – Procarbazine is taken daily and I was given a supply to take away with me.
- C – CCNU was given to me in tablet form on the first day.
- V – Vincristine was given intravenously over thirty minutes on the first day.

Hooked up to the drip, I looked around at the others sitting in the ward. It was all quite matter-of-fact: nobody looked that sick, some old, some young, some bald and most not. My father later described it as being like a group of women at a hair salon having their hair blow-dried. Just chatting and reading, it was all very relaxed.

The side effects were minimal. An anti-sickness tablet, Domperidone, combated the nausea and vomiting. I had to avoid certain foods that may have caused an allergic reaction, but it was really only the fatigue that I noticed. I adopted the policy that if I ate something that made me feel sick, I stopped eating it. If I felt tired, I rested. If I felt good, I went outside and got some fresh air. You don't have to be bedridden!

I really was a walking pharmacy though. On top of my anti-convulsant medication and chemo, I was still taking the hormone replacement drugs, hydrocortisone, thyroxin and testosterone. I was also taking Dexamethasone, a steroid that helps to prevent brain swelling. It is taken in conjunction with Lanspoprazole, which prevents stomach ulcers caused by some of the steroids I was on. A side-effect of Dexamethasone is that is does make you very hungry, and, combined with its other side effect, constipation, it creates some quality toilet time! The daily ritual of drug-taking was just a part of the process, but I did feel sometimes that the only reason I was standing upright was because of medication.

19 November, 2003

Each treatment was a process I had to go through, and eventually I would beat this damned thing. It might take time, but I would be buggered if I was going to die from this illness. If one treatment didn't get it, the next one would. It wasn't about prolonging my life but rather about the lengthy course of treatment required to deal with an aggressive cancer. No longer a case of *if* I would beat my tumour, but *when!* A few years battling an illness, out of a lifetime of say eighty years, was nothing, and would always be a good story to tell the grandchildren!

As the seven months of chemotherapy drew to a close, the partial paralysis I had suffered began to disappear, until my full movement was restored. My tumour responded well to chemo and, after a series of clear routine MRI scans in 2004, I had confirmation that my tumour had finally gone, for good.

Epilogue

Cam Fulljames is still instructing new pilots on the systems of the jet aircraft that his airline operates. Although not flying, he is nevertheless immersed in the business he adores. Working in the operational side of an airline has opened up many exciting opportunities in the aviation industry for Cam. His ambition is to be a flight operations director of a major U.K. airline and he hopes to one day own his own light aircraft, and fly for pleasure.

He continues to live happily in Edinburgh with his beloved Sarah and they are planning a Scottish wedding in the summer of 2006. He still takes occasional trips back to New Zealand to check in with his family and friends.

In keeping with his desire to "give something back," Cam continues to have contact with young people with terminal illness and is a financial supporter of Imperial Cancer Research, U.K.

It is Cam's hope that this book might bring a glimmer of reassurance and support to anyone suffering from a terminal illness, as well as to their friends and family.

To this day, Cam has not had another seizure.

Postscript

I am often asked how I feel within myself about what has happened to me. My answer is always this: "I have always rationalised my illness by saying that if brain tumours really do occur randomly, then far rather I dealt with it than some wee kiddie or someone in less of a position to cope than I was. It would be very easy to crawl up into the foetal position and cry yourself to sleep, but I don't think that's in our nature as human beings. The will to survive, rise to the challenge and the will to live is strong in all of us; it just needs to be coaxed out sometimes. The love and support from friends, family and colleagues has a tremendous impact on us to kick-start and maintain our determination to beat our adversity. It must be remembered that there is always somebody worse off than ourselves. The parent that has lost their family in a car accident or the person dying from AIDS. Their pain and suffering must never play second fiddle to your own."

You get on, get going and make the best of it!

Contacts & Information

One of the reasons I wanted to publish my diary and experiences of cancer was to help other people with a similar plight. I believe that information and the right support – or at least knowing where to go for it - can make a huge difference in recovery, and that there could be more information out there for people to tap into.

The following people, organisations and references outline the resources that helped me empower myself through knowledge, and to gain a sense of control at a time when I needed it most. They are listed here in the hope that they can be of similar assistance to others when they need it most.

Internet

The Web is an invaluable resource. You should attempt to find out as much as you can about your illness. There are, of course, many websites, so be specific when using your search engine. Entering the type of tumour you have is a good start, e.g., astrocytoma.

Try: www.tbts.org - run by The Brain Tumor Society or
www.braintumor.org – run by the National Brain Tumor Foundation U.S.A.

Books

Information booklets produced by hospitals or support groups are a very good resource. Brain Tumour Action (BTA) in the United Kingdom publishes two booklets in particular that I found most helpful. They are entitled *Living with a Brain Tumour* and *Radiotherapy for Brain Tumours*.

Stay clear of medical books, as they are difficult to navigate and tend to include life expectancy statistics that can be a bit frightening.

To get yourself into the right frame of mind, I highly recommend *Love, Medicine and Miracles* by Bernie Seigel.

Nutrition

Considering your nutritional requirements is particularly important during chemotherapy. Given the negative effect on your liver and kidney and the risk of anaemia, I recommend:

1. Drink plenty of water
2. Eat fresh, raw, organic vegetables
3. Eat plenty of fresh fruit for the vitamin C and antioxidant value
4. I also took Life Pak! four tablets taken daily containing essential minerals and vitamins and antioxidants for the body. Life Pak is available from Pharmanex – www.europe.pharmanex.com

Treatments

Apart from the tried-and-tested radiotherapy and chemotherapy, there are many treatments being developed all the time, and it is worth discussing any new treatment with your consultant, certainly if you would like to be involved in any trials.

Of note, a strain of the common cold sore virus has been found effective in attacking malignant cells while leaving healthy brain cells unharmed.

Shark cartilage can be effective. When inserted into the brain, it draws away the blood that is feeding the tumour's growth.

Scientists have also discovered the gene responsible for triggering the brain tumour medulloblastoma in children.

For those with an open mind who might consider natural healing, I highly recommend visiting Harry Oldfield's website (www.electrocrystal.com). Harry, who is based in London, has had huge successes in the treatment of breast cancer.

Stereotactic Radiotherapy

Performed in the UK in London and Sheffield and the USA. Check out gramma.knife via your web search.

Erressor

A new drug developed in Japan. Although not yet approved in the UK, it must be worth checking out.

Consultants

A professor of neurology who has global contacts, looks for other opinions, has empathy and is someone that you can trust, is essential. You don't have to accept the first diagnosis or treatment plan. Seek a second opinion if your physician has not done so.

The following heath professionals looked after me and are very approachable. They may be contacted through the Western General Hospital, Edinburgh.

Professor Ian Whittle
Department for Clinical Neurosciences
Western General Hospital
Crewe Road South
Edinburgh
EH4 2XU

Dr. Anna Gregor
Oncology Department
Western General Hospital
Crewe Road South
Edinburgh
EH4 2XU

Support Groups

Consult the hospital that is treating you for contact details. But remember, the support groups are not for everyone and are only as good as the people running them.

For young people and their parents, the Maggie Centre, with branches located across the United Kingdom, is superb.

I am always available if you just want to chat: ctulljames@hotmail.com

Above all, remember that you are not alone.

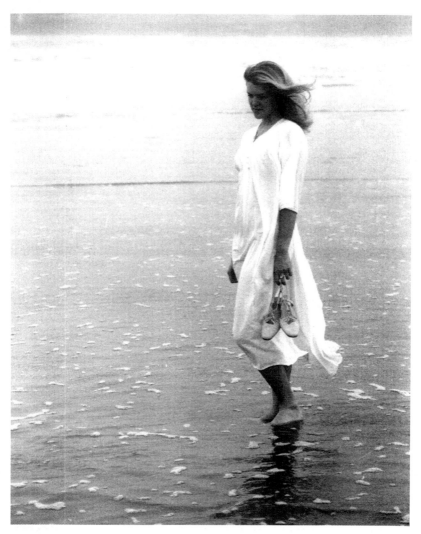

'Sarah my Angel'
I took this photograph of Sarah during
my photography course.

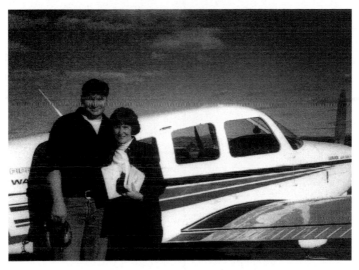

Taking Mum for a flight, having just graduated from my commercial pilot's course.

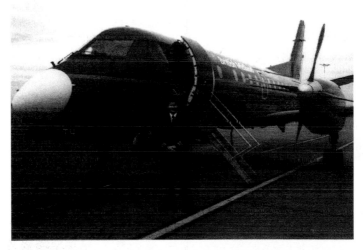

My first flight as an airline pilot, with British Midland.

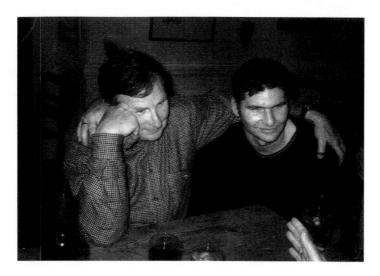

Dad, my mate, and me!

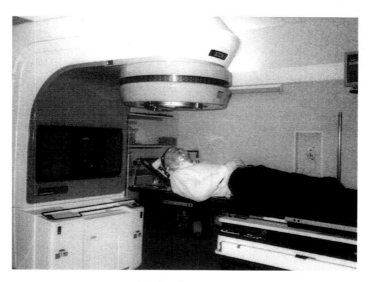

Radiotherapy.

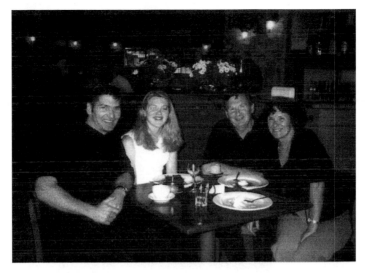

Sarah and I with Mum and Dad on holiday in New Zealand.

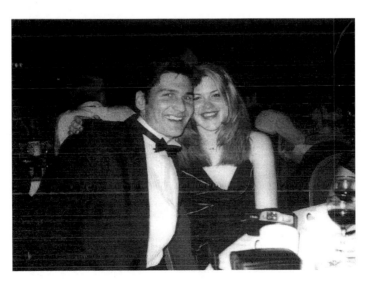

Sarah's Medical Ball, April 2000.

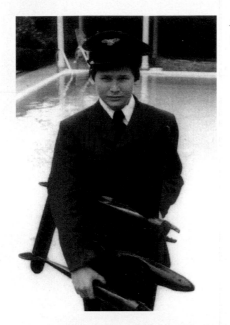

At seven years of age I took aviation very seriously!

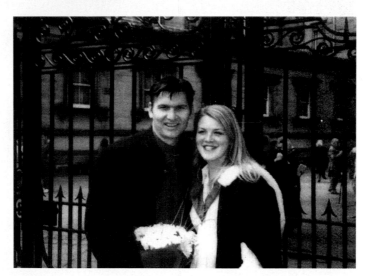

Sarah's graduation.